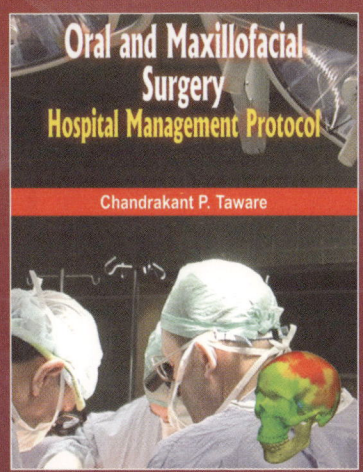

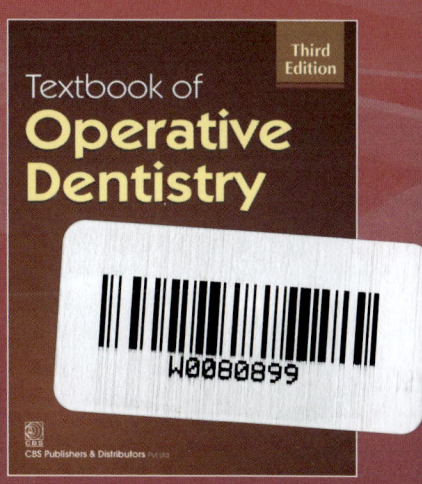

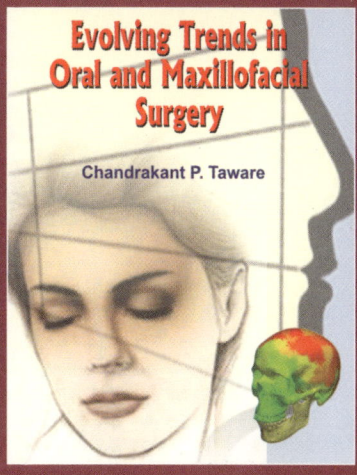

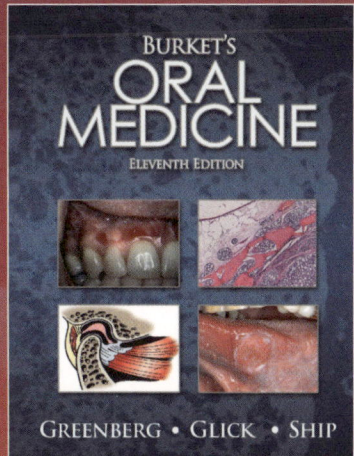

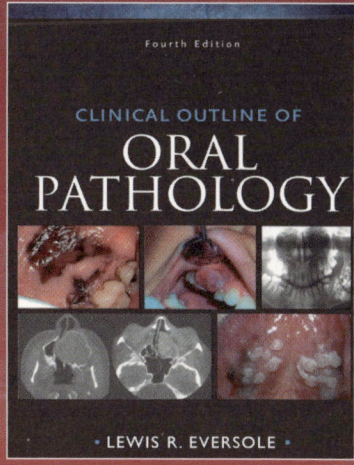

Temporomandibular Joint

IMAGING

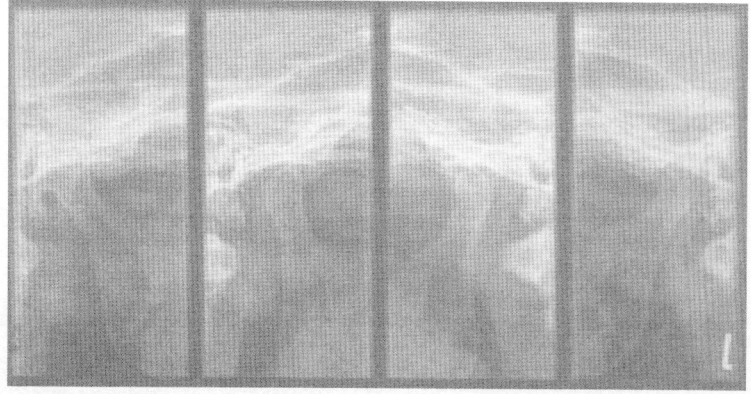

Temporomandibular Joint
IMAGING

Rahul Srivastava MDS
Senior Lecturer, Department of Oral Medicine and Radiology
Rama Dental College, Hospital and Research Centre
Lakhanpur, Kanpur, UP

Parvathi Devi MDS
Professor and Head, Department of Oral Medicine and Radiology
Teerthankar Mahaveer Dental College and Research Centre
Moradabad, UP

Bhuvan Jyoti MDS, PGDHHM
Dental Surgeon and Consultant in Oral Medicine and Radiology
Department of Dental Surgery
Ranchi Institute of Neuro-Psychiatry and Allied Sciences
Kanke, Ranchi, Jharkhand

CBS Publishers & Distributors Pvt Ltd
New Delhi • Bengaluru • Chennai • Kochi • Mumbai • Pune
Hyderabad • Kolkata • Nagpur • Patna • Vijayawada

Temporomandibular Joint
IMAGING

ISBN: 978-81-239-2397-0

Copyright © Authors and Publishers

First Edition: 2014

Published by Satish Kumar Jain for
CBS Publishers & Distributors Pvt Ltd

4819/XI Prahlad Street, 24 Ansari Road, Daryaganj, New Delhi 110 002, India.
Ph: 23289259, 23266861, 23266867   Website: www.cbspd.com
Fax: 011-23243014   e-mail: delhi@cbspd.com; cbspubs@airtelmail.in.

Corporate Office: 204 FIE, Industrial Area, Patparganj, Delhi 110 092
Ph: 4934 4934   Fax: 4934 4935   e-mail: publishing@cbspd.com; publicity@cbspd.com

Branches

- **Bengaluru:** Seema House 2975, 17th Cross, K.R. Road, Banasankari 2nd Stage, Bengaluru 560 070, Karnataka
  Ph: +91-80-26771678/79   Fax: +91-80-26771680   e-mail: bangalore@cbspd.com
- **Chennai:** 20, West Park Road, Shenoy Nagar, Chennai 600 030, Tamil Nadu
  Ph: +91-44-26260666, 26208620   Fax: +91-44-42032115   e-mail: chennai@cbspd.com
- **Kochi:** 36/14 Kalluvilakam, Lissie Hospital Road, Kochi 682 018, Kerala
  Ph: +91-484-4059061/65   Fax: +91-484-4059065   e-mail: kochi@cbspd.com
- **Mumbai:** 83-C, Dr E Moses Road, Worli, Mumbai-400018, Maharashtra
  Ph: +91-22-24902340/41   Fax: +91-22-24902342   e-mail: mumbai@cbspd.com
- **Pune:** Bhuruk Prestige, Sr. No. 52/12/2+1+3/2 Narhe, Haveli (Near Katraj-Dehu Road Bypass), Pune 411 041, Maharashtra
  Ph: +91-20-64704058/59, 32392277   Fax: +91-20-24300160   e-mail: pune@cbspd.com

Representatives

- **Hyderabad** 0-9885175004
- **Nagpur** 0-9021734563
- **Kolkata** 0-9831437309, 0-9051152362
- **Patna** 0-9334159340
- **Vijayawada** 0-9000660880

Printed at: HT Media Ltd., Noida

Preface

There has been a long-standing demand from dental students which would help them to understand the basic techniques for temporomandibular joint (TMJ) imaging. Temporomandibular joint imaging is an adjunct to the clinical examination and provides useful information about the joint components. Temporomandibular joint imaging provides information about the status and function of the joint that helps in establishing a definitive diagnosis. When selecting a TMJ imaging technique, the clinician must determine what type of information is needed from imaging study and whether that information will affect patient management. Knowing the diagnostic accuracy of imaging modality is essential for its clinical use. The accuracy of tomography, arthrography, computed tomography (CT) and magnetic resonance (MR) imaging has been investigated in several studies, all techniques have demonstrated relatively high accuracy in determining osseous conditions and disk position; however, MR imaging has the highest accuracy and demonstrates both joint structures and the soft tissues surrounding the joint.

We have tried our level best to include almost all imaging techniques. We hope that this book will reduce the burden of dental students in learning the imaging assessment of TMJ. We will feel amply rewarded if the book satisfies the readers and will be grateful to them if they provide us the feedback to improve text further.

Rahul Srivastava
Parvathi Devi
Bhuvan Jyoti

Acknowledgments

Every author owes a great deal to others and we are not an exception. First and the foremost, we bow in gratitude to the Almighty for His blessings.

We dedicate this book to Late KC Srivastava whose advice and expertise continue to be greatly missed.

We wish to thank Mr YN Arjuna, Senior Director at CBS Publishers & Distributors for his continuous help and patience in the production of this book.

Finally to our family members, Sushila Devi, AJ Bihari, M Bihari, Janardhan Amarnath, Usha, Swati Swadesh, Jeevan, Vineeta and the lovely children Manya, Harshini, Tanya, Sanskaar and Tanay, for their understanding and constant support.

Rahul Srivastava
Parvathi Devi
Bhuvan Jyoti

Contents

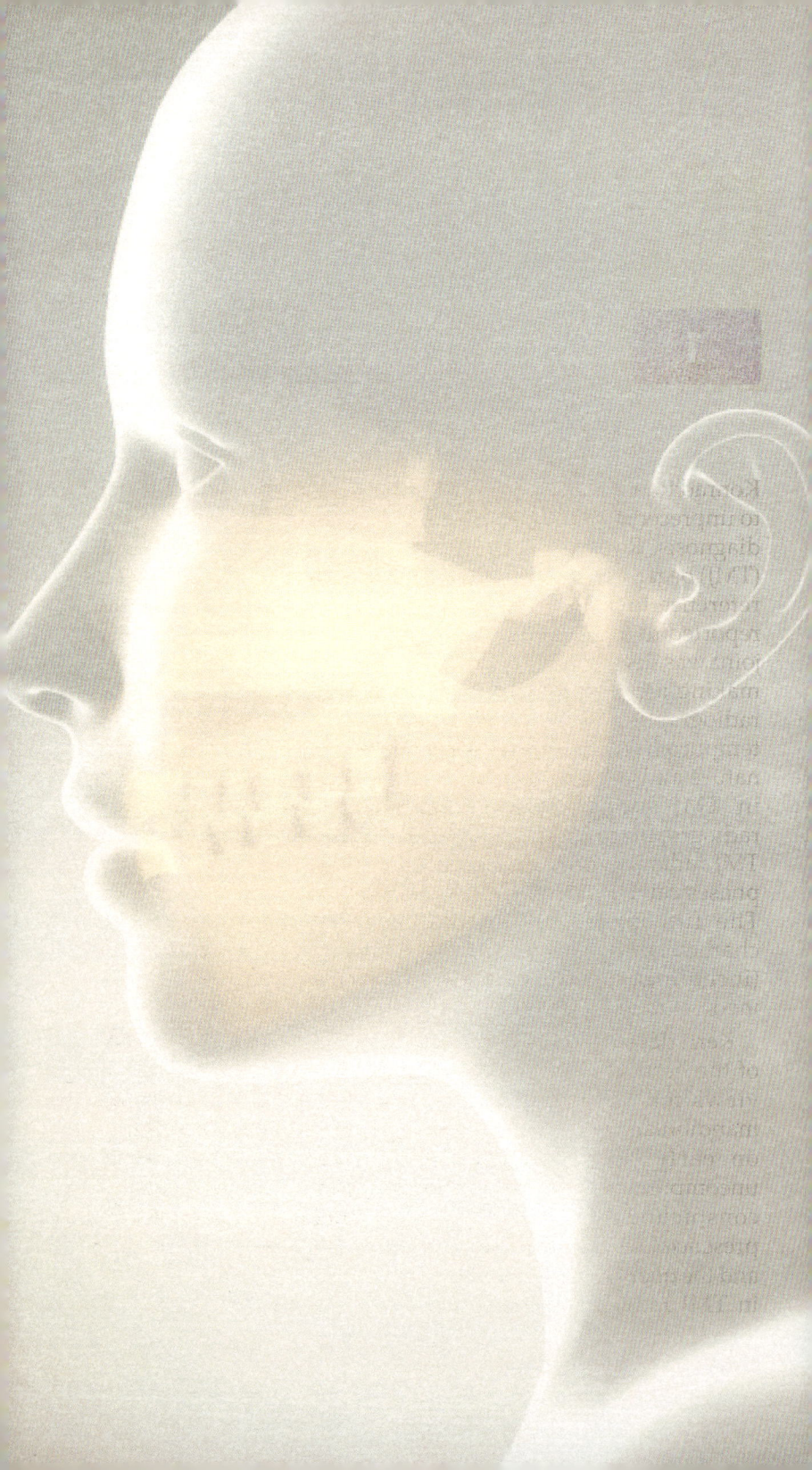

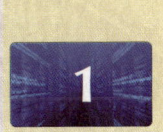

Introduction

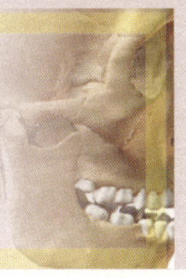

Konrad Roentgen's discovery of X-rays in 1895 opened the door to unprecedented exploitation of a new technology for medical diagnosis. Roentgenographs of the temporomandibular joint (TMJ) began appearing in the early 1900s. Blair made the earliest reference to TMJ radiograms in discussing a case that was reported to the St. Louis Medical Society in 1910. Usually one joint was disordered, but occasionally both were involved and making a correct diagnosis was complicated by inadequate radiographs. Murphy complained that "the skiagrams of the temporomandibular joint do not shed much light upon the nature and extent of an injury to the joint." Clearly, advances in TMJ surgery demanded the advancement of TMJ radiographic techniques. A review of the literature shows that TMJ radiography evolved in a cyclical fashion. Three distinct phases can be identified over a period of more than 70 years. The first phase, lasting approximately 30 years, was characterized by relatively intense activity in transcranial (including stereoscopic) TMJ radiography, principally by medical radiologists.

Kern developed a technique for making stereoscopic views of the head. He recommended that dental surgeons use such views for "impacted molars and arthritic changes in the mandibular joints". Bishop provided an important perspective on early TMJ radiography: "TMJ radiograms are … uncomplimentary to the roentgenologist because… they are conspicuous by their absence or unconvincing by their presence." As the techniques of TMJ radiography were refined and the quality of TMJ radiographs improved, a broader interest in TMJ radiographs developed, particularly on the part of dentists. Lindblom devised a technique for registering the position of the mandibular condyle within the glenoid fossa to obtain accurate transcranial radiographs. Essentially this was the beginning of what are called corrected TMJ radiographs; the technique of directing the central X-ray beam along a path consistent with the morphology of certain joint structures. Usually the condylar long axis, but Highley used the summit of the articular eminence and Maves the glenoid fossa for their respective anatomic landmarks for corrected TMJ radiographs. Highley designed a rather precise cephalostat that held the head in a 20 degree rotation with 8 degrees of lateral tipping. Maves apparently had a cephalostat that he intended to market to dentists and he gave notice of intent. Maves made an interesting reference to the radiographic documentation of condylar position before and after placing dental occlusal splints. After nearly 50 years this concept is still applied to TMJ therapy.

At the 1948 meeting of the American Dental Association, Updegrave outlined his improved technique for transcranial TMJ projections and made specific recommendations for advancing the quality, safety and reproducibility of TMJ transcranial radiograms. One of his chief purposes was to introduce a technique that could be easily adopted by dentists using ordinary dental X-ray equipment. This was an important step toward greater involvement of dentists in joint imaging, since up to this time TMJ radiography was chiefly the domain of medical radiologists. However, Updegrave's technique (using a +15 degree angled board) did not differ markedly from those of Kern, Bishop, or Sproull. Over the next 20 years laminagraphic, fluoroscopic and cineradiographic TMJ studies were published, but radiographic research did not increase significantly until the 1970s.

The first reported study of TMJ computed tomography in the United States was done by Suarez and others in 1980. This work gave examples of different joint conditions and presented correlated autopsy tissue sections to support the radiographic findings. Beginning in 1981 the number of TMJ CT papers nearly doubled each year through 1985, after which they declined sharply because of the emergence of magnetic resonance imaging. Although most of the clinical TMJ CT studies originated in the United States, investigations were underway in Italy, West Germany, the Netherlands, Egypt, Israel, Scandinavia and the People's Republic of China. As search progressed, it became apparent that computed tomography had some limitations in visualizing the disk. As is often the case with new techniques and modalities, imaging applications had surged ahead of clinical practice. The early published reports of MRI investigations of the temporomandibular joint appeared in 1984 and 1985. Caution is needed, however, because basic research must be conducted into the MRI signal characteristic of normal and abnormal joint tissues and the imaging accuracies of various systems and pulsing sequences must be established. Research project in progress should more clearly define the role of MRI in the continuum of imaging choices that face medical and dental radiologists. The development of TMJ arthroscopy paralleled that of computed tomography and magnetic resonance imaging. For arthroscopy the question awaiting an answer is what would contribute to TMJ diagnosis compared to conventional and advanced imaging modalities? The role of clinical management and TMJ radiology now appear to be reversed from what they were 70 years ago. Diagnostic imaging technology is developing rapidly and is ahead (hopefully only temporarily) not only of surgery, but also of dentist's ability to effectively manage many TMJ disorders. Currently the greatest research and clinical opportunities lie in the coherent application of advanced imaging modalities to the basic investigations of TMJ disorders. Regrettably, because of the present confusion about TMJ pathology and patient management, skeptics within dentistry may pose the greatest obstruction to such efforts.

BIBLIOGRAPHY

1. Christiansen EL, Thompson JR. A book on Temporomandibular Joint Imaging. St.Lovie 1990 Mosby.
2. Helms CA, Richardson ML, Moon KL, Ware WH. Nuclear magnetic resonance imaging of temporomandibular joint: Preliminary observations. J Craniomand Prac 1984, 2;3:219–24.
3. Katzberg RW, Schenck JF, Roberts D, et al. Magnetic resonance imaging of temporomandibular joint. Oral Surg. 1985;59:332–5.
4. Roberts D, Schenck J F Joseph P, et al. Temporomandibular joint magnetic resonance imaging. Radiology 1985;155:829–30.

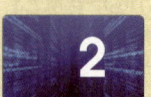

Temporomandibular Joint

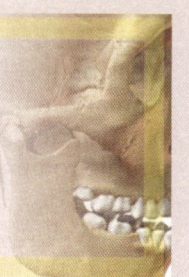

Articulation of the lower jaw to skull is achieved by bilateral articulation between condyles of mandible and temporal bone of the skull. Temporomandibular joint, also known as ginglymoarthrodial (diarthrosis) joint, is a synovial joint and is one of the most complex joints in the body. It provides hinging movement in one plane and therefore can be considered as a ginglimoid joint. At the same time it also provides gliding movements, which classifies it as an arthrodial joint. Hence the name, *Ginglymoarthrodial*. It is a so called secondary joint (Gaupp, 1911) because it developed separately and not as a modification of a primary joint (Dabelow, 1928).

DEVELOPMENT OF TEMPOROMANDIBULAR JOINT

Upper and lower jaw bones as well as temporal bones derived from the mesenchyme develop from neural crest cells during the 4th week of embryonic development. Out of this mesenchyme, pharyngeal arches develop in the head and neck area and they participate in facial development. After 4–5 weeks of development, the stomodeum is surrounded by an even numbered mandibular process (ventral part of the first pharyngeal arch), even numbered maxillary process (dorsal part of the first pharyngeal arch), and by a frontal process from above.

In the mandibular process, Meckel's cartilage is formed. The tympanic and mandibular process of Meckel's cartilage is completely developed in the 16th week of embryonic development. The thickened posterior ending of the tympanic cartilage is the primordial cartilage called the malleus. Malleus in direct contact with the primordial cartilage called incus by means of a flat articulation plane. From the 8th until the 16th week of development, the primordial cartilages function as the primary temporomandibular or malleoincudal joint; auditory ossicles develop from the latter. This joint can perform only simple rotation or buccal movements, which appear in the 8th week of development. All these movements are important for the development of condylar cartilage. Later, the malleus is separated from Meckel's cartilage and ossified to become the middle ear ossicle. Meckel's cartilage is important for the topographic organization and differentiation of the facial structures during embryonic and fetal development.

The mandibular primary growth center starts developing from the 12th week in the mandibular process of Meckel's cartilage. It has a morphogenetic role in lower jaw development because it marks the beginning of the intramembranous ossification of the mandible.

The volume of Meckel's cartilage decreases after the 18th week and later it disappears during mandibular ossification. Meckel's cartilage is replaced by the body of the mandible and secondary condylar cartilage. A characteristic of mandibular development is bone derivation from the mesenchyme by intramembranous ossification, laterally from Meckel's cartilage, while the development of carrot-shaped condylar cartilage is placed posteriorly. TMJ development takes place mostly between the 7th and 20th week of intrauterine life and a particularly sensitive period is morphogenesis between the 7th and 11th week. A particular feature of TMJ development compared to other joints in the human body is mutual approximation of the initial condylar and temporal base (blastema). There are three stages in TMJ development: Blastemic stage (7 to 8th week; development of the condyles, articular fossa, articular disk and capsule), cavitation (9 to 11th week; beginning of lower joint space development and condylar chondrogenesis), and maturation stage (after the 12th week). The tiny eminences on the ascending ramus of the mandible are the bases of the condylar and the coronoid processes. In the 9th week, chondrogenesis begins from the mesenchyme cells, laterally from Meckel's cartilage, in the middle of the condylar blastema. In the 10th week, the condylar head and the entire conical condyle are apically surrounded by the lower jaw body, which is ossified intramembraneously. Enchondral ossification of the condylar cartilage in the anterior part begins in the 17th week and after the 20th week the cartilaginous form of the condyle is present only on the surface. The existence of temporal bone is visible from the 8th and 9th week. It is situated above the most distal part of Meckel's cartilage and above the base of the malleus and incus auditory ossicles. During the 8th week, the zygomatic process of the temporal bone is ossified. In the 10th week, there is medial thickening of the disk with mildly pronounced concave contours. In the period of the 11th and 12th week, the articular fossa can be concave, convex or completely flat. The articular fossa spreads cranially from the condyle in anterior direction and from the 12th week it has a concave shape.

The extension of the articular eminence and postglenoid process appears after the 26th week. After the 7th week, mesenchymal thickening is visible, positioned craniolaterally from the future condyle, out of which the articular disk develops.

Due to the forming of articular spaces, the articular disk is thinner in the middle section, which later creates a characteristic biconcave shape. From the 12th week, it is in its permanent position between the temporal bone and the condyle.

Its cartilaginous structure is clearly visible between the 15th and 20th week. The mesenchymal development of the articular capsule starts in the 8th week and stretches from the squamous part of the temporal bone towards the articular disk and the condyle. In the 11th week, the capsule is positioned between the zygomatic arch of the temporal bone and the condyle and it is attached to the outer portion of the articular disk. The upper and lower articular spaces develop from several cracks in the thickened mesenchyme, from which the condyle, the articular disk and the capsule develop. Lower articular space starts developing earlier, but slower than the upper one, in the 9th week, and follows the condylar base shape. The upper articular space starts forming in the 11th week between the zygomatic process of the temporal bone and the articular disk. It grows laterally and anteriorly between the 12th and 16th week of development. The articular spaces are disproportionate until the 26th week. The secondary TMJ is fully developed after the

14th week of intrauterine growth, anteriorly from the otic capsule, and after the 16th week it assumes the primary joint function. The ossified parts of the primary joint (malleus and incus) become part of the middle ear. Only two other rudimentary otomandibular ligaments remain to be developed, without functional significance. The discomalleolar ligament connects the anterior malleolar ligaments and ends in the posterior threads of the articular disk. The malleomandibular ligament is a remainder of Meckel's cartilage and it goes through the tympanosquamous fissure.

ANATOMY OF TEMPOROMANDIBULAR JOINT

Articular Surfaces

The upper articular surface is formed by following parts of temporal bone

1. Articular eminence
2. Anterior part of mandibular fossa.

Inferior articular surface is formed by head of mandible (Fig. 2.1).

Glenoid Fossa

Mandibular condyle articulates at the base of cranium with squamous portion of temporal bone. It is a concave fossa, limited:

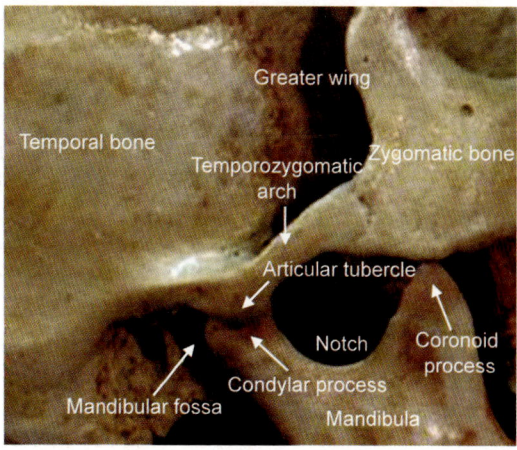

Fig. 2.1: Articular surfaces

Posteriorly: By squamotympanic fissure.
Medially: By spine of the sphenoid.
Laterally: Root of zygomatic process of temporal bone.
Anteriorly: Ridge of articular eminence.

Degree of convexity of the articular eminence is highly variable, but important because steepness of this surface dictates pathway of condyle when the mandible is positioned anteriorly. The posterior root of the mandibular fossa is quite thin indicating that this area of the temporal bone is not designed to sustain heavy forces.

Mandibular Condyle

1. Condyle is the portion of the mandible that articulates with cranium around which movement occurs.
2. From anterior view it has a medial and lateral projection called poles—medial pole and lateral pole.
3. Medial pole is generally more prominent than lateral pole.
4. Condyle is convex, wider mediolateral than anterioposterior. Length (mediolateral) 15–20 mm and (anterioposterior) 8–10 mm.
5. Actual articulating surface of condyle extends both anteriorly and posteriorly to most superior aspect of the condyle. Posterior articulating surface is greater than anterior articulating surface.
6. The articulating surface of condyle is quite convex anteroposteriorly and only slightly convex mediolaterally.

Articular Disc

1. Collagenous fibrous tissue of variable thickness is called articular disc. It is also called meniscus.
2. It is fibrous in nature.
3. It is situated between articular surface of joint and divides the joint into the upper compartment and lower compartment.
4. Articular disc is composed of dense fibrous connective tissue, for the most part is devoid of any blood vessels or nerve fibers.
5. Extreme periphery of the disc, however, is slightly innervated.

6. In the sagittal plane, it can be divided into three regions according to thickness: Intermediate, posterior, anterior. Central area is thinnest and called intermediate zone. Posterior zone is slightly thicker than anterior border.

In normal joint articular surface of the condyle is located on the intermediate zone of the disc bordered by thicker anterior and posterior region. Central thinner component separates the anterior slope of the condyle from the slope articular eminence. Thickened posterior position occupies gap between condyle and floor of glenoid fossa. From the anterior view, disc is generally thicker medially than laterally which corresponds to the increased space between condyle and articular fossa towards medial side joint. Precise shape of the disc is determined by morphology of condyle and mandibular fossa. During movement disc is somewhat flexible and can adapt to functional demands of articular surfaces.

Anteriorly disk is divided into two lamellars. Upper one runs forward to fuse with capsule and periosteum in the anterior slope of eminence. Lower runs down to attach to the front of neck of the condyle. In between the foot of the disc which merges either with capsule or upper surface of muscle fiber constituting upper component of superior head of lateral pterygoid muscle. Articular disc is attached posteriorly to a region of loose connective tissue that is highly vascularised and innervated and is known as retrodiscal tissue or posterior attachment. Superiorly it is bordered by a lamina of connective tissue that contains many elastic fibers (superior retrodiscal lamina). Superior retrodiscal lamina attaches the articular disc posteriorly to tympanic plate.

Lower Lamina

Lower border of the retrodiscal lamina attaches the inferior border of posterior edge of the disc to the posterior margin of articular surface of condyle.

Inferior retrodiscal lamina is composed of collagenous fibers unlike elastic fibers of superior retrodiscal lamina. Remaining body of retrodiscal tissue is attached posteriorly to a large nervous plexus which fills with blood as condyle moves forward. The superior and inferior attachment of the anterior region of disc capsular ligament surrounds most of the joint.

The superior attachment is to the anterior margin of the articular surface of the temporal bone. The inferior attachment is to the anterior margin of the articular surface of the condyle. Both of these anterior attachments are composed of collagenous fibers.

Upper and Lower Cavity

Articular disc is attached to capsular ligament not only anteriorly and posteriorly, but also medially and laterally. This attachment divides the joint into lower and upper cavities (Fig. 2.2). The upper or superior cavity is bordered by the mandibular fossa and the superior surface of the disc. The lower or inferior cavity is bordered by mandibular condyle and inferior surface of disc.

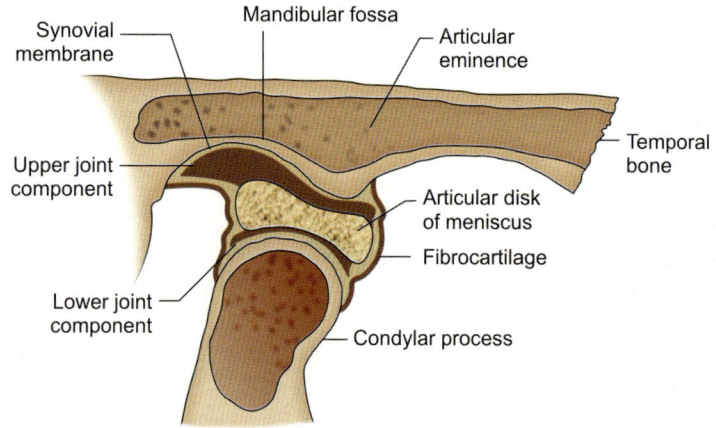

Fig. 2.2: The upper and lower cavities

Capsule and Synovial Membrane

Surrounding the joint is a fibrous capsule which extends from margins of glenoid fossa including articular eminence anteriorly to envelop head of condyle before fusing inferiorly with periosteum of the condylar process. The capsule thus encloses a joint cavity which is divided into two compartments by a flattened fibrous disk which, except at its posterior margin, is attached for the most part peripherally to the capsule.

Synovial Membrane

Internal surface of capsule is lined by a synovial membrane. Finger like projections or villi of synovial membrane occur in anterior and posterior limit of joints to accommodate the movement of capsule. Synovial membrane consists of two layers, cellular intima resting on a vascular sub-intima which in turn blends with fibrous capsule.

The subintima is a loose connective tissue containing blood vessels, scattered fibroblast, macrophages, mast cells, fat cells and some elastic fibers which prevent folding of membrane. The intimal layer consists of cells embedded in an amorphous fiber free intercellular matrix varying in thickness from 1 to 4 cells.

Cells of this layer are essentially an intermingling of fibroblasts like type B cells and macrophages like type A cells. Type A cells exhibit phagocytic properties and synthesize hyaluronate found in synovial fluid. Type B cells is thought to add protein to fluid.

Synovial Fluid

Synovial fluid is a dialysate of plasma to which is added some protein and sodium hyaluronate as a result of activity of fibroblast like cells. Its total volume is approximately 1 ml. Increased muscular loading across joint surface or biochemical alteration in the synovial fluid leads to loss of viscosity and increased frictional resistance.

Specialized endothelial cells that form a synovial lining surround the internal surfaces of cavities. This lining, along with a specialized synovial fringe located at the anterior border of retrodiscal tissues, produces synovial fluid, which fills both joint cavities. Thus, temporomandibular joint is referred to as synovial joint. Because articular surfaces of the joint are non vascular, synovial fluids acts as a medium for providing metabolic requirements to these tissues. Free and rapid exchange exists between vessels of capsule, the synovial fluid and the articular tissues. Synovial fluid also serves as a lubricant between articular surfaces during function. Synovial fluid lubricates the articular surface by two mechanisms.

    a. Boundary lubrication.
    b. Weeping lubrication.

Boundary Lubrication

Occurs when joint is moved and synovial fluid is forced from one area of cavity into another. Synovial fluid located in the border or recess areas is forced on the articular surface thus providing lubrication. It prevents friction in moving joint and is the primary mechanism of joint lubrication.

Weeping Lubrication

It is the ability of articular surfaces to absorb a small amount of synovial fluid. Weeping lubrication helps to eliminate friction in the compressed, but not in moving joint. It only helps to remove a small amount of friction.

Relations of TMJ

- **Laterally:** Skin and facial.
  Parotid gland.
  Temporal branch of facial nerve.
- **Medially:** Tympanic plate.
  Spine of sphenoid with upper end of sphenomandibular ligament attached to it.
  Auriculotemporal and chorda tympanic nerve.
  Middle meningeal artery.
- **Anteriorly:** Lateral pterygoid.
  Masseteric nerve and vessel.
- **Posteriorly:** Superficial temporal vessel.
  Auriculotemporal nerve.
- **Superiorly:** Middle cranial fossa.
  Middle meningeal vessel.
- **Inferiorly:** Maxillary artery and vein.

Ligaments

Ligaments play an important role in protecting the structure. Ligaments of the joint are made up of collagenous connective tissues that have particular length and do not stretch. If extensive forces are applied to a ligament whether suddenly or over a prolonged period of time ligament can be elongated. Ligaments do not enter actively into joint function rather they act as passive restraining device to limit and restrict border movements.

Three functional ligaments

- Collateral ligament
- Capsular ligament
- Temporomandibular ligament

Two accessory ligaments

- Sphenomandibular
- Stylomandibular

A. Collateral Ligament

It attaches to the medial and lateral borders of the articular disc to the poles of condyle. They are commonly called discal ligaments:

- **Medial discal ligament:** Attaches medial edge of the disc to the medial pole of condyle.
- **Lateral discal ligament:** Attaches lateral edge of disc to lateral pole of condyle.

Discal ligaments are true ligaments composed of collagenous connective tissue fibers, therefore, they do not stretch. They function to restrict movement of disc away from condyle. Attachment of the discal ligaments permits disc to be rotated anteriorly and posteriorly on the articular surface of the condyle. Ligaments are responsible for the hinging movement of TMJ which occurs between condyle and articular disc.

B. Capsular Ligament

Entire TMJ is surrounded and encompassed by capsular ligament. Fibers of capsular ligament are attached superiorly to the temporal bone along the borders of articular surfaces of mandibular fossa and articular eminence. Inferiorly the fibers of capsular ligament attach to the neck of condyle. Capsular ligament acts to resist any medial lateral or inferior forces that tend to separate or dislocate the articular surfaces. Significant function of capsular ligament is to encompass the joint thus retaining synovial fluid.

C. Temporomandibular Ligament

Temporomandibular ligament is composed of an outer oblique portion and inner horizontal portion.

Inner Horizontal Portion

It extends from the outer surface of articular tubercle and zygomatic process, posteriorly and horizontally to the lateral pole of condyle and posterior part of articular disc.

Inner horizontal portion of the temporomandibular ligament limits posterior movement of the condyle and disc. When force is applied to the mandible it displaces the condyle posteriorly. This portion of the ligament becomes tight and prevents the condyle from moving into posterior region of mandibular fossa and protects the retrodiscal tissue from trauma caused by posterior displacement of condyle. Also protects lateral pterygoid muscle from over lengthening or extension. Effectiveness of this ligament is demonstrated during the cases of extreme force on mandible. In such cases neck of condyle will fracture before the condyle enters middle cranial fossa.

Outer Oblique Portion

It extends from the outer surface or articular tubercle and zygomatic process postero inferiorly to the outer surface of condylar neck. Oblique portion of the temporomandibular ligament resists excessive dropping condyle, therefore, limiting extent of mouth opening. During initial phase of opening the condyle can rotate around a fixed point until temporomandibular ligament becomes tight as its point of insertion on the neck of condyle is rotated posteriorly. When the ligament is taut the neck of condyle cannot rotate further. If jaw is opened still wider a distinct change in opening movement will occur which represents change from rotation of the condyle around a fixed point to movement forward and down the articular eminence, this change is brought about by tightening of temporomandibular ligament. This unique feature of temporomandibular ligament which limits rotational opening is found only in human. In the erect postural position and with a vertically placed vertebral column continued rotational opening movement would cause mandible to impinge on the vital submandibular and retro-mandibular structures of the neck. Outer oblique portion of the temporomandibular ligament functions to resist this impingement.

Accessory Ligament

A. Sphenomandibular Ligament

Arises from spine of sphenoid and extends downwards to a small bony prominence on the medial surface of ramus of mandible called the lingula.

B. Stylomandibular Ligament

It arises from styloid process and extends downwards and forward to the angle and posterior border of ramus of mandible. It limits excessive protrusive movement of mandible, it becomes taut when mandible is protracted, but is most relaxed when the mandible is opened (Fig. 2.3).

Innervation of Temporomandibular Joint

Temporomandibular joint is innervated by same nerve (trigeminal nerve) that provides motor and sensory innervation to the muscles that control it. Innervation is provided by auriculotemporal nerve as it leaves mandibular nerve behind the joint. Ascends laterally and superiorly to wrap around the

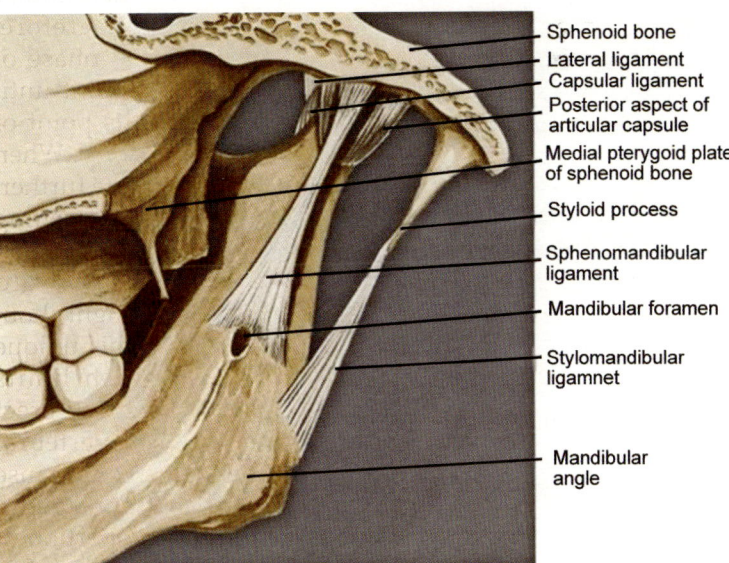

Sphenoid bone
Lateral ligament
Capsular ligament
Posterior aspect of articular capsule
Medial pterygoid plate of sphenoid bone
Styloid process
Sphenomandibular ligament
Mandibular foramen
Stylomandibular ligamnet
Mandibular angle

Fig. 2.3: Stylomandibular ligaments

posterior region of the joint. Deep temporal and masseteric nerves provide additional innervations.

Vascularisation of Temporomandibular Joint

Temporomandibular joint is richly supplied by a variety of vessels that surround it. Predominantly vessels are superficial temporal artery and internal maxillary artery. Condyle receives its vascular supply through its narrow spaces by way of the inferior alveolar artery and by way of feeder vessels that enter directly into condylar head both anteriorly and posteriorly from larger vessels.

BIBLIOGRAPHY

1. Avery JK. Essentials of oral histology and embryology: a clinical approach. 2nd ed. St. Louis: Mosby, 2000:29–41, 156–64.
2. Avery JK. Development of cartilage and bones of the craniofacial skeleton. In: Avery JK, editor. Oral development and histology. 3rd ed. Stuttgart-New York: Thieme, 2001:44–59.
3. BD Chaurasia's Human Anatomy. pp 150–52.
4. Bontemps C, Cannistr a C, Hanneck e V, Mich el P, Fonzi L, Bar bet JP. The first appearance of Meckel's cartilage in the fetus. Bull Group Int Rech Sci Stomatol Odontol 2001;43:94–9.
5. George A Zarb. Temporomandibular Joints and Masticatory Muscle disorders Chapter 2. pp 48–65.
6. Gola R, Chossegros C, Cheynet F. Oto-mandibular ligaments: disco-mallear and malleo-mandibular ligaments. Rev Stomatol Chir Maxillofac 1997;98:66–71.
7. Jeffery P. Okeson. Management of Temporomandibular Disorders and Occlusions 5th edition.pp 3–28.
8. Lee SK, Kim YS , Oh HS, Ya ng KH, Kim EC, Chi JG. Prenatal development of the human mandible. Anat Rec 2001;263:314–25.
9. Martinez G, Calta biano C, Leonar di R, Calta biano M. Histomor-phology of secondary cartilage in human fetal mandibles. Minerva Stomatol 1997;46:39–43.
10. Merida-Velasco JR, Rodriguez-Vazq uez JF, Merida-Velasco JA, Sa nch ez-Montesinos I, Espin-Ferra J, Jimenez-Collado J. Development of the human temporomandibular joint. Anat Rec 1999:255:20–33.
11. Radlanski RJ, Sepadi L, Bontsch ev NE . Development of the human temporomandibular joint. Computeraided 3D-reconstructions. Eur J Oral Sci 1999;107:25–34.
12. Sadler TW. Langman's medical embryology. 11th ed. Philadelphia: Lippincott Williams and Wilkins, 2010.

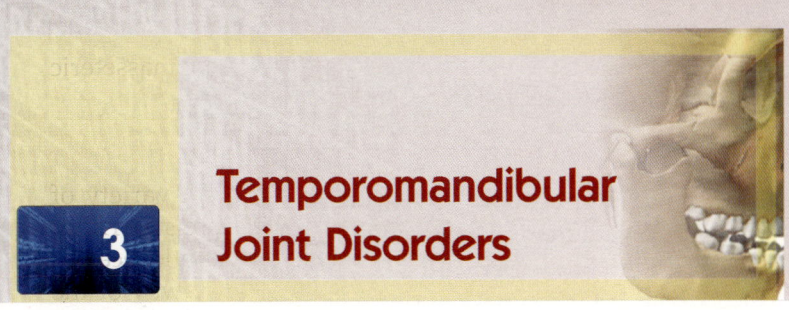

Temporomandibular Joint Disorders

3

Temporomandibular disorders (TMD) is a collective term embracing all the problems relating to the TMJ and related musculoskeletal structures. It is an umbrella term which combines those with true pathology of the temporomandibular joint and those with involvement of the muscles of mastication (myofascial pain dysfunction). The classification of TMD is listed below.

TEMPOROMANDIBULAR JOINT AND RELATED MUSCULOSKELETAL DISORDERS

(Approved by American Society of Temporomandibular Joint Surgeons)

I. Intra-articular (Intracapsular) Pathology

A. Articular capsule
1. Displacement
2. Deformity
3. Adhesions
4. Degeneration
5. Injury
6. Perforation
7. Anomalous development

B. Disc attachments
1. Inflammation
2. Injury (laceration, hematoma, contusion)
3. Perforation
4. Fibrosis
5. Adhesions

C. Synovium
1. Inflammation/effusion
2. Injury
3. Adhesions
4. Synovial hypertrophy/hyperplasia
5. Granulomatous inflammation
6. Infection
7. Arthritides (rheumatoid, degenerative)
8. Synovial chondromatosis
9. Neoplasia

D. Articular fibrocartilage
1. Hypertrophy/hyperplasia
2. Generation
   a. Fissuring
   b. Fibrillation
   c. Blistering
   d. Erosion

E. Mandibular condyle and glenoid fossa
1. Osteoarthritis (osteoarthrosis, degenerative joint disease)
2. Avascular necrosis (osteonecrosis)
3. Resorption
4. Hypertrophy
5. Fibrous and bony ankylosis
6. Implant arthropathy
7. Fracture/dislocations

II. Extra-articular (Extracapsular) Pathology

A. Musculoskeletal
1. Bone (Temporal, Mandible, Styloid)
   a. Anomalous development (hypoplasia, hypertrophy, malformation, ankylosis)
   b. Fracture
   c. Metabolic disease
   d. Systemic inflammatory disease (connective tissue/arthritides)
   e. Infection
   f. Dysplasia
   g. Neoplasia

2. Masticatory muscles and tendons
   a. Anomalous development
   b. Injury
   c. Inflammation
   d. Hypertrophy
   e. Atrophy
   f. Fibrosis, contracture
   g. Metabolic disease
   h. Infection
   i. Dysplasias
   j. Neoplasia
   k. Fibromyalgia

B. Central Nervous System/Peripheral Nervous System

1. Reflex sympathetic dystrophy

In 1972, Farrar proposed a classification that contemplates eight dimensions within the global concept of dysfunction.

Hyperactivity of the masticatory muscles, capsulitis and synovitis, rupture or distension of the capsular ligaments, anterior disc displacement, muscle in coordination and reduction of the mandibular movement range secondary to degenerative joint disease.

Classification of Temporomandibular Joint Disorders. Axis I (Physical aspects) (Dworkin and LeResche, 1992)

Group I: Muscle disorders
   I.a. Myofascial pain
   I.b. Myofascial pain with limitations in aperture

Group II: Disc displacement
   II.a. Disc displacement with reduction
   II.b. Disc displacement without reduction and no limitations in aperture
   II.c. Disc displacement without reduction and with limitations in aperture

Group III: Arthralgia, arthritis, arthrosis
   III.a. Arthralgia
   III.b. Osteoarthritis of the TMJ
   III.c. Osteoarthrosis of the TMJ

Etiology of Temporomandibular Disorders

Three main groups of etiologic factors were proposed:
1. Anatomic (including the occlusion and the joints)
2. Neuromuscular
3. Psychologic

Etiologic Factors

Trauma, emotional stress, orthopedic instability, and muscle hyperactivity were implicated as significant components.

Predisposing Factors

A. Systemic (general health),
B. Psychologic (personality, behaviour), or
C. Structural (occlusion, joint).

Initiating (or precipitating) factors usually involve trauma, overloading, or parafunction.

Perpetuating (or sustaining) factors often include behavioural, social and emotional problems and other forms of stress and general health.

Trauma

Two general types of trauma need to be considered:
1. Macro trauma
2. Micro trauma.

A force that exceeds normal functional loading can lead to injury of the affected structures.

Macro trauma is any sudden force to the joint that causes structural alterations. Macro trauma can also occur when the teeth are together (closed mouth trauma) or can produce a sudden displacement of the condyle within the fossa (open mouth trauma).

Occlusion

Several activities of the masticatory system seem to have no functional purpose and are therefore referred to as parafunctions. Occlusal parafunctions include bruxism (teeth grinding or clenching), lip biting, thumb-sucking, and abnormal posturing of the jaw. Bruxism has been suggested as an initiating or perpetuating factor in a certain subgroup of temporomandibular disorders.

General Health

Several epidemiologic studies have shown that individuals with impaired general health tend to suffer more frequent and severe TMD signs and symptoms than healthy people. The most common systemic conditions are rheumatologic diseases.

Psychosocial Factors (Axis II—Mental Aspects)

The role of psychologic disturbances in the etiology of TMD also is controversial. It is widely recognized that psychological factors may be involved in the pain perception process. Although the etiology of TMD has not been established, psychological factors have been implicated in the predisposition, initiation, and perpetuation of TMD.

Congenital Anomalies

The TMJ can be affected by several developmental anomalies, embryonic and postembryonic. Congenital anomalies of the TMJ are rare. Dr. Clark suggests that recent evidence (Rugh and Ohrbach, 1988) leads us to believe that stress, parafunctional habits and abnormal loading may amplify the pain of this disorder.

SYMPTOMS AND SIGNS OF TEMPOROMANDIBULAR JOINT DISORDERS

Temporomandibular disorders (TMD) are according to the Guidelines of the American Academy of Orofacial Pain, 'a collective term embracing a number of clinical problems that involve the masticatory musculature, the temporomandibular joints and associated structures, or both'. More than 100 diseases can affect the musculoskeletal system, and many of these may also involve the TMJ. Some of these diseases are relatively common and well known, such as osteoarthrosis/osteoarthritis, rheumatoid arthritis while others such as infectious and metabolic diseases are rare. Levitt, Lundeen, and McKinney prepared a scale for clinicians of all specialties that consider the influence of psychological variables and the presence of problems not related to TMJ. In Norway, Heloe collected anamnestic TMJ data from 246 individuals, 25 yrs of age. Of these young people 20% said they had experienced joint clicking or crepitation, and 8% of these felt pain while opening the mouth wide, chewing, yawning, or talking.

Symptoms and Signs

1. Pain, headache, and muscle spasms.
2. Clicking, snapping, popping, grating noises in the TMJ.
3. Dizziness and possible nausea.
4. Earache, ringing in the ears (tinnitus), a fullness or pressure backlog in the ear.
5. Pain or burning sensation of tongue.
6. Partial or complete inability to open the mouth.
7. Limited range of function of the mandible in one or more directions, with or without pain.
8. Tender areas on face and head where palpation elicits painful response either in the area palpated or to a referred pain area.
9. Neck aches and backaches.

Symptoms of TMDs occur in approximately 6 to 12 percent of the adult population or approximately ten million individuals in the United States. It is estimated that 17,800,000 workdays are lost each year for every 100,000,000 full-time working adults in the United States due to disabling TMDs.

The epidemiologic predilection of TMDs in women is striking. In the general population, TMDs are two times more prevalent in women than in men, whereas in patient populations these diseases have a female-to-male preponderance as high as 10:1. Furthermore, unlike similar diseases of other joints, which also have a greater female predilection, but occur postmenopausally, a large proportion of women with TMDs are between eighteen and forty-five years of age. The reasons for this marked sexual dimorphism and age distribution remain unclear.

Rheumatic Diseases

Helenius et al found in their study that patients suffering from the various rheumatic diseases exhibits higher prevalence of stomatognathic problems and radiographic evidence of TMJ destruction than the matched controls. The patients with mixed connective tissue disorder exhibited lower prevalence of individual symptoms, abnormal findings on examination, and erosions than the other patients.

Crum and Loiselle studied 26 patients with ankylosing spondylitis and they found that symptoms associated with ankylosing spondylitis were bilateral pain and tenderness in the TMJ region, with limited mouth opening.

Myofascial Pain and Dysfunction

Costen believed that patients with edentulous mouths and a marked overbite were more likely to develop symptoms. Schwartz differentiated between generic TMJ syndrome, and myofascial pain dysfunction syndrome. Laskin gave the psychophysiologic theory of myofascial pain dysfunction. In 1988, Reynolds challenged the concept of a TMJ pain syndrome, stating that it should be discarded in favor of more specific muscular and/or articular disorders.

It was shown by Murphy and Adams that the radiographic reports of the temporomandibular joint in patients with myofascial pain are almost always unremarkable. Usually no signs of degenerative joint disease are found, nor are there any indirect radiographic signs of disc displacement, such as condylar malpositioning or joint space widening, with conventional X-ray studies.

Disc Dislocation

The term internal derangement historically has referred to joints (not just TMJ) that do not function smoothly. Now it is believed that the term internal derangement is used to denote articular disc displacement. Normally the disc is placed between the condyle and the articular fossa and facilitates condylar movements. Depending on how the disc may interfere with condylar movement, the joint may click or pop, onomatopoiec terms for different intensities of the same phenomenon. If the disc interferes with but does not block condylar translation, the condition is assumed to be displacement with reduction, because the condyle negotiates its way onto the disc. If the disc prevents condylar translation, the condition is called displacement without reduction, known as closed lock. Further the disc displacement with or without reduction can be lateral, medial, anterolateral, anteromedial, anterior, rotational and rarely posterior disc displacement. Farrar and McCarty define disc displacement as anterior displacement of disc associated with posterior-superior displacement of the condyle in closed jaw position. They also refer to disc displacement as dysfunctional centric relation. Hellsing and Holmlund do not recognize anterior disc displacement as an abnormal disc position, maintaining that different disc positions are merely variations of normal. Malpositioning of disc from normal to abnormal position usually is accompanied by joint sounds such as clicking or prominent popping. Noisy joints with displaced and reducing disc are often painful, but not always. Detectable clicking, popping can be a sign of a dislocated, reducing articular disc. When clicking, popping or both are noted, the mandible usually translates a normal distance (40 to 55 mm), but with a rapid perturbation toward the affected side. The perturbation coincides with the click. Not all deranged joints click or pop. Some osseous conditions may mimic disc dislocations. If the condyle encounters a bony irregularity on the articular surfaces accompanying noises may be mistaken for a malpositioned disc. Dislocated disc rarely click at the same point when the jaws are opened and closed. Clicking caused by a bony irregularity occurs at the same point in the translatory cycle. Disc dislocations may become an important factor in the degeneration of the osseous components of the temporomandibular joint. Katzberg and others found radiographic evidence of degenerative changes in 22% of patients they followed.

Westesson, Bronstein and Liedberg found that the extent of soft and hard tissue change was related to the degree of anterior disc malpositioning. When the disc was completely anterior to the condyle, irregularities were found in the articular surfaces in 65% of cases. As the disc was less and less anterior to the condyle, disc deformations and osseous changes dropped and were around 31%.

BIBLIOGRAPHY

1. Christiansen EL, Thompson JR. A book on Temporomandibular Joint Imaging. St.Lovie 1990 Mosby.
2. Crum RJ, Loiselle RJ. Temporomandibular joint symptoms and ankylosing spondylitis. J Am Dent Assoc 1971;83:630–3.

3. Guidelines for Diagnosis and Management of Disorders Involving the TMJ and Related Musculoskeletal Structures approved by American Society of Temporomandibular Joint Surgeons II.

4. Hellsing G, Holmlund A. Development of anterior disc displacement in the temporomandibular joint: an autopsy study. J Prosthet Dent 1985;53:397–401.

5. Katzberg RW, Keith DA, Guralnick WC, et al. Internal derangements and arthritis of temporomandibular joint. Radiology 1983;146:107–12.

6. L Miia, J Helenius, Hallikainen D, Helenius I, et al. Clinical and radiographic findings of the temporomandibular joint in patients with various rheumatic diseases. A case control study. Oral Surg Oral Med Oral Pathol Endod 2005;99:455–63.

7. Rafael Poveda Roda, et al. Review of temporomandibular joint pathology. Part I: Classification, epidemiology and risk factors. Med Oral Patol Oral Cir Bucal 2007;12:E 292–8.

8. S. Baskan, A. Zengýngul, Temporomandibular Joint Disorders and Approaches Biotechnol and Biotechnol. Eq.20/2006/2 ;151–5.

9. Wadhwa S, Kapila S. TMJ Disorders: Future Innovations in Diagnostics and Therapeutics. Journal of Dental Education 2008; 72(8):930–47.

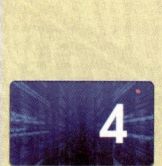

Temporomandibular Joint Imaging

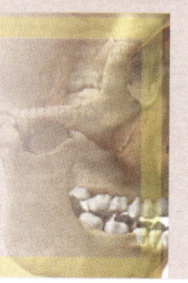

4

INTRODUCTION

The need for imaging of the TMJ should be established on the basis of selection criteria. Selection criteria represent those clinical signs and symptoms that suggest that a radiographic examination would contribute to the proper diagnosis and care of the patient. They provide a rationale for selecting among the various imaging modalities, with the goal of obtaining the necessary diagnostic information without unnecessary patient expense and radiation exposure.

The most appropriate imaging procedures are those that provide new information that will influence patient care. Selection of an examination is influenced by many, sometimes competing factors. The decision should be made after considering the history and clinical findings, clinical diagnosis, cost of examination, amount of radiation exposure and results of prior examinations, as well as tentative treatment plan and expected outcome.

Imaging of temporomandibular joints and associated structures is necessary to establish the presence or absence of pathology and stage of disease in order to select appropriate treatment, assist in prognosis and assess patient response to therapy.

The type of imaging technique selected depends on:
A. The specific clinical problem.
B. Whether imaging of hard and soft tissues is desired.
C. The amount of diagnostic information available from a particular imaging modality.
D. The cost of the examination.
E. The radiation dose.

In most cases the imaging protocol begins with hard tissue imaging to evaluate the osseous contours, the positional relationship of the condyle and fossa and the range of motion, although a combination of imaging techniques may be indicated. Soft tissue imaging is indicated when information about disc position, morphology, or integrity is needed or to image abnormalities in the muscles or surrounding tissues.

Classification

The hard tissues, soft tissues or a combination of both TMJ structures can be seen in an image form. For hard tissue assessment (i.e. bony changes, condylar position) the following imaging techniques can be considered.

Hard Tissue Imaging

1. Transcranial projection
2. Transpharyngeal projection
3. Transorbital projection
4. Submentovertex projection
5. Reverse Towne's projection
6. Dental panoramic tomogram
7. Conventional tomography
8. Computed tomography

For evaluation of soft tissue components of TMJ (such as articular disc), the following imaging techniques can be considered.

Soft Tissue Imaging

1. Arthrography
2. Magnetic resonance imaging
3. Ultrasound

Plain Film Radiography

The term plain film radiographs refers to radiographs made with a stationary X-ray source and film. Plain films of TMJ depict only the mineralized part of the joint and do not reveal nonmineralized cartilage and soft tissues. In addition superimposition of adjacent anatomic structures makes visualization of all parts of the joint difficult, although imaging the joint from multiple angles helps overcome this limitation.

The most useful plain film radiographs of the TMJ appear to be oblique transcranial, the transmaxillary and the submento-vertex views. Each of these is projected approximately 90 degrees to the other two. The transpharyngeal view is some-times used as an alternative to the transcranial projection. Disc position cannot be determined from any of these techniques.

Transcranial Projection

The lateral oblique transcranial projection directs the X-ray beam approximately parallel to the long axis of the condyle. The 15 to 25 degree positive vertical (caudal) angle reveals the lateral aspect of the joint as the bony contour seen on the radiograph. The central and medial portions of the joint are projected downward, superimposing on the rest of the condylar process.

Area of Joint

- Glenoid fossa
- Articular eminence
- Joint space
- Condylar head

Main Indications

- For the study of the condyle in the glenoid fossa.
- For assessment of joint space for partial or complete obliteration of joint space as in case of ankylosis or effusion.
- To study the bony contour of the superior surface of the condyle and the articular eminence for presence of erosions and/or sclerosis.
- For any bony growth in the anterosuperior surface of the condyle.
- To investigate the range and degree of movements of the condyle.
- To investigate the size and position of the disc; this can be inferred indirectly from the relative positions of the bony elements of the joints.

Limitation

The neck of the condyle is not seen because of superimposition of surrounding structures.

Film Position

The cassette is placed flat against the patient's ear and centered over the temporomandibular joint of interest, against the facial skin parallel to the sagittal plane.

Position of Patient

The patients head is adjusted so that the sagittal plane is vertical.

The ala tragus line is parallel to the floor (Fig. 4.1).

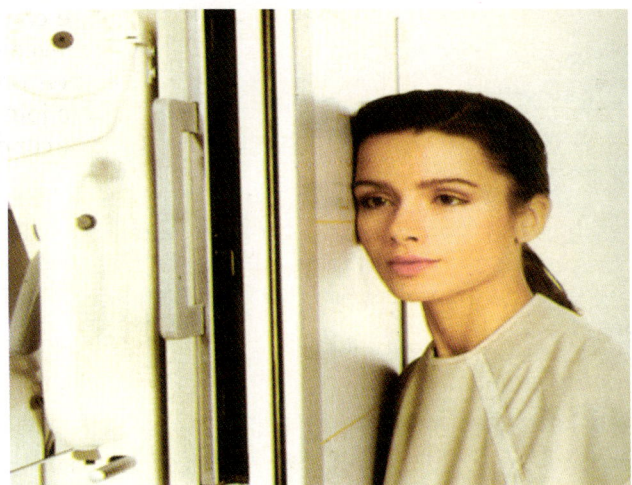

Fig. 4.1: Positioning of the patient

This view is taken with the patient's mouth in following positions:

Open mouth

Closed mouth.

CENTRAL RAYS

The point of entry is different according to the technique used.

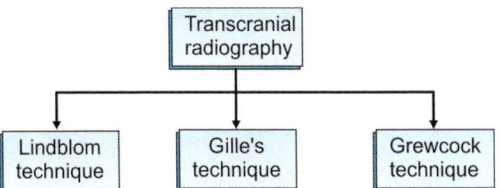

Lindblom Technique or Postauricular

Point of entry of the central ray is ½ inch behind and 2 inches above the external auditory meatus (Fig. 4.2).

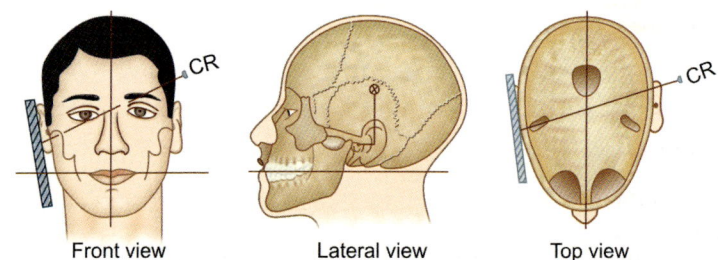

Front view   Lateral view   Top view

Fig. 4.2: Central ray entered is ½ inch behind and 2 inches above the external auditory meatus

According to Lindblom the central ray should be directed from posteriorly so that it passes along the long axis of the condyle (the medial pole of the condyle is more posterior to the lateral pole).

Grewcock Technique

The central ray enters through a point 2 inches above the external auditory meatus perpendicular to occlusal plane (Fig. 4.3).

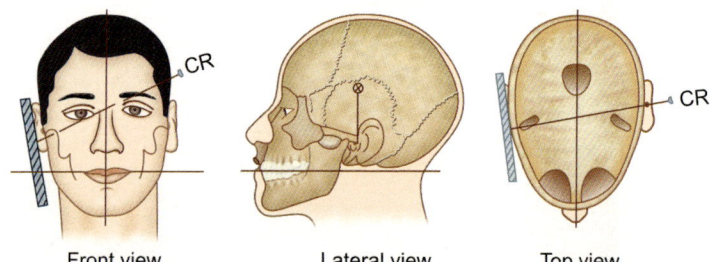

Front view   Lateral view   Top view

Fig. 4.3: Direction of entry of the central ray in Grewcock technique

Gille's Technique

The central ray enters through a point ½ inch anterior and 2 inches above the external auditory meatus. Parallel and perpendicular to occlusal plane (Fig. 4.4).

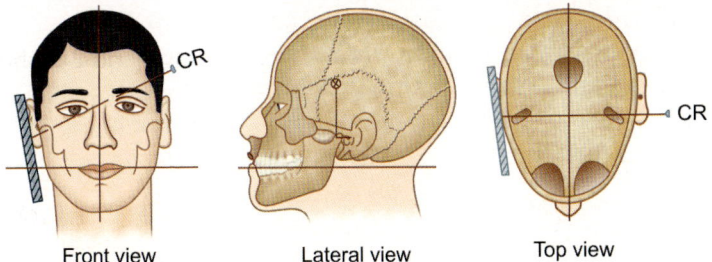

Front view   Lateral view   Top view

Fig. 4.4: Direction of entry of the central ray in Gille's approach

In all the three techniques the central ray is directed caudally at angle of –20° to +25°.

The point of exit is through the TM joint of interest.

Exposure Parameters

KVp–70   mA–07   Seconds–1.5

Diagnostic Information

Closed View

The size of the joint space. This provides indirect information about the position and shape of the disc.

Joint space refers to the radiolucent zone between the condylar head and glenoid fossa, which includes the disc and the upper and lower anatomical joint spaces (Fig. 4.5).

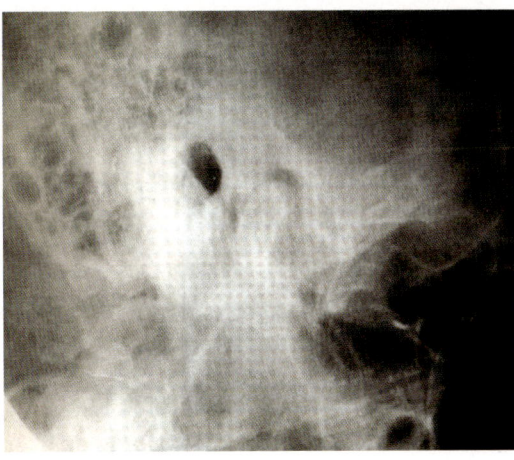

Fig. 4.5: Transcranial view

- The position of the head of the condyle within the fossa.
- The shape and condition of the glenoid fossa and the articular eminence (on the lateral aspect).
- The shape of the head of the condyle and the condition of the articular surface (on the lateral aspect).
- A comparison of both sides.

Open View

- The range and type of movement of the condyle.
- A comparison of the degree of movement on both sides.

The glenoid fossa is clearly seen in the transcranial projection. The lateral one fourth to one third of the condyle is best visualized with the transcranial projection because the X-ray beam is tangential to the superior surface of the lateral pole. The greater the positive vertical angle of the beam's central ray, the greater the separation between the projected lateral and medial condylar poles. However, vertical angles greater than 20 degrees significantly distort the joint structures on open mouth views. It is well documented that approximately half of all osseous changes occur in the lateral joint. The best radiographic detail available in a plain film technique is given by microfocal magnification which, according to Murphy and others, provides improved resolution, greater perception of bone detail, decreased noise, and greater diagnostic value. The magnified examination is still only a transcranial radiograph.

ASSESSMENT OF JOINT SPACE AND CONDYLAR POSITION

Transcranial projections may give a false impression of the envelope of condylar joint space because of the modality's emphasis on the lateral joint structures. Pullinger and Hollender compared the adequacy of transcranial projections and linear tomograms in determining the condylar position. They found agreement between the two methods in 60% of cases, but were mildly critical about the lateral oblique transcranial projection for monitoring small changes in condylar position relative to the tomogram.

Aquilino and others evaluated the accuracy of three different transcranial TMJ radiographic records of condylar position and joint space dimension. They also evaluated how reliably observers determined condylar position and joint space dimensions from the radiographs. They concluded that the classification of condylar position is not the same at different sagittal location within a TMJ, skull position and radiographic projection must be identical if joint space measurements from serial radiographs are to be compared, the actual joint space dimensions and the anatomic anterior/posterior position of the condyles in the glenoid fossa cannot be accurately recorded by the radiographic techniques used in the investigation and condyle/fossa relationships cannot be classified reliably by subjective evaluation of TMJ radiographs.

Preti and Fava compared transcranial projections to fluoroscopy for accurately displaying condylar position. They concluded that fluoroscopy gives better results.

Curious as to why a relatively high proportion of transcranial projections were noninterpretable, they began a second phase of their study, using computed tomograms of the same patient sample.

They found that superimposition on transcranial projections played a minor role and that the principal difficulty lay in the morphologic profile of the posterior condylar border. They reasoned that this resulted from poor visualization of the glenoid outline, most probably caused by the petrotympanic fissure, which interrupts the posterior wall of the glenoid fossa.

Disc Displacement

Carl Dixon and others compared two transcranial radiographic methods in diagnosing TMJ anterior disc displacement with arthrography. Both transcranial radiographic methods could only accurately predict the presence of an anteriorly displaced disc in a range of 26 to 56% of the time. The methods were more valuable in correctly identifying joints that were free of disease.

Detection of Osseous Disease

Transcranial projections are superior to most other plain film techniques for detecting osseous diseases of the condyle, but not of temporal component. The earliest arthritic changes tend to occur on the crest of the articular eminence significantly.

Mongini contrasted plain films and tomograms in 30 patients with TMJ symptoms. He noted that the degenerative changes could not be detected clearly with transcranial TMJ projections. Omnell and Petersson compared the information from standardized and individualized transcranial projections to that yielded by tomograms in a study of the temporomandibular joints of 30 patients. They found that tomography revealed the greatest number of structural changes, followed by individualized technique (71% as effective) and the standardized technique (28% as effective).

Transmaxillary Projection/Transorbital Projection

Also known as Zimmer/Transmaxillary projection.

Area of Joint
- Anterior view of the TMJ
- Entire mediolateral dimension of the articular eminence
- Condylar head
- Condylar neck

Main Indications
- For mediolateral displacement of the condyle in condylar neck fractures.
- To evaluate the relation of the condyle in the mediolateral plane.
- To see the superior surface of the condyle for osteophytes, etc.
- A useful adjuvant to transcranial and transpharyngeal projections in the diagnosis of the degenerative changes or other anomalies.

Technique and Positioning
- The film cassette is placed behind the patient's head.
- The patient's head is tilted downward 10 degrees so that the canthomeatal line is horizontal (Fig. 4.6).

The X-ray beam is directed from the front of the patient downward approximately 10 degrees and laterally approximately 30 degrees through the ipsilateral orbit and centered over the TMJ of interest (Fig. 4.7).

The patient is asked to open his mouth as far as comfortable, or as an alternative, protrudes the mandible, thereby positioning the condyle at the summit of the articular eminence,

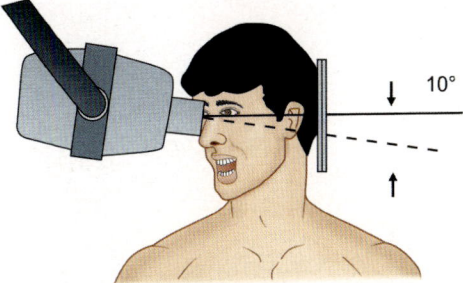

Fig. 4.6: The direction of entry of the central beam in transorbital projection

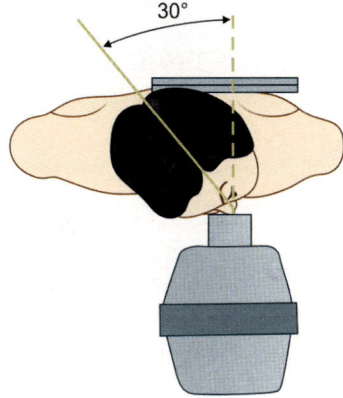

Fig. 4.7: 30 degrees angulation of the X-ray beam

thus avoiding superimposition of the articular eminence or skull base on the condyle (Fig. 4.8).

The route of X-ray beam's central ray through the maxillary sinus to the condyle gives this technique its name. With this projection the condyle may be superimposed on the articular eminence, particularly if the patient cannot open his/her mouth easily or if it is open too widely. This projection does not show the fossa, but the erosive condylar changes are seen nearly twice as well as with either the transcranial or transpharyngeal view.

Transpharyngeal Projection

This view is effective for demonstrating destructive changes of the condyle, but less valuable for productive changes. It may

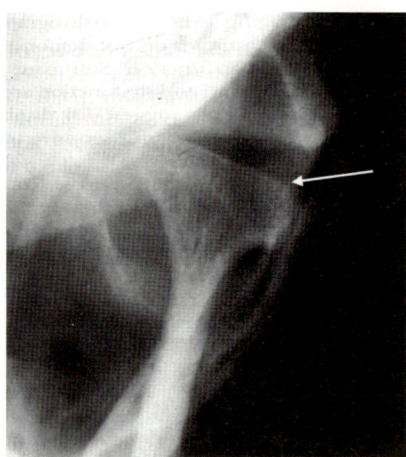

Fig. 4.8: Transorbital view

also be of value in diagnosing fractures of the condylar neck. Information about the temporal component of the joint is not available.

Also known as **Infracranial/Parma or Mac Queen Projection.**

Area of the Joint

Lateral view of
- Condylar head and neck
- Articular surface

Main Indications

- To investigate the presence of joint disease, particularly osteoarthritis and rheumatoid arthritis.
- To investigate pathological conditions affecting the condylar head, including cysts or tumors.
- To observe any change in the neck and head of the condyle as in case of fractures.
- For developmental anomalies like condylar hyperplasia or hypoplasia.
- For elongated styloid process as in Eagle's syndrome.

Technique and Positioning

- The patient holds the cassette against the side of the face over the TMJ of interest. The film and the sagittal plane of the head are parallel. The patient's mouth is open and a bite block is inserted for stability.

• The X-ray tube head is positioned in front of the opposite condyle and beneath the zygomatic arch. It is aimed through the sigmoid notch, slightly posteriorly, across the pharynx at the condyle under investigation.

• Usually this view is taken for both the condyles to allow comparison.

• The central ray is oriented superiorly 5–10 degrees and posteriorly approximately 10 degrees, centered over the TMJ of interest (Fig. 4.9 and 4.10).

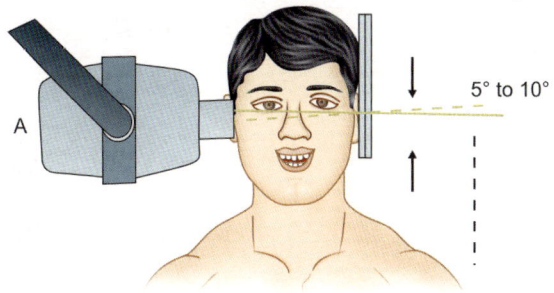

Fig. 4.9: Horizontal angulation of the central beam

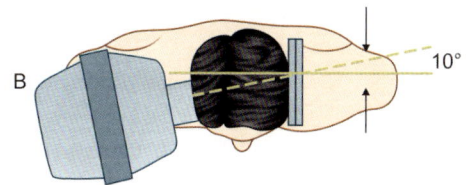

Fig. 4.10: 10 degrees posterior angulation of the central beam

Exposure Parameters

Kvp–70   mA–07   Seconds–0.8

Diagnostic Information

• The shape of the head of condyle and the condition of the articular surface from the lateral aspect.

• A comparison of both the condylar heads.

Limitations

- The condyle is seen obliquely.
- Minute bony alterations on the anterior condylar surface will not be projected.

In the transpharyngeal or infracranial projection the fossa is not clearly seen. If the mouth is not adequately open, the condyle may be superimposed on the articular eminence. The osteophytes are revealed equally by transpharyngeal and transcranial projections. The anterolateral part of the condyle is best seen in this view. If the angulation of the condylar axis is low, the condylar profile is better seen with the transpharyngeal projection than with the transcranial projection. The radiation dose is high because of the short target to film distance.

Submentovertex Projection

It is also called the *base or full axial projection.* This projection shows the base of the skull, sphenoidal sinuses and facial skeleton from below. The submental-vertex view (SMV) reveals the base of the skull with the beam projected through the chin region parallel to the posterior border of the ascending ramus. A cephalostat is helpful in obtaining a symmetrical head position, thus minimizing distortion.

Indications

The main clinical indications includes

- Destructive/expansive lesions affecting the palate, pterygoid region or base of the skull
- Investigation of the sphenoidal sinus.
- Assessment of the thickness (mediolateral) of the posterior part of the mandible before osteotomy.
- Fracture of the zygomatic arches—to show these thin bones, the SMV is taken with reduced exposure factors.

Technique and Positioning
Image Receptor and Patient Placement

The image receptor is positioned parallel to patient's transverse plane and perpendicular to the midsagittal and coronal planes. To achieve this, the patient's neck is extended backward as far as possible, with the canthomeatal line forming a 10° angle with the image receptor (Fig. 4.11).

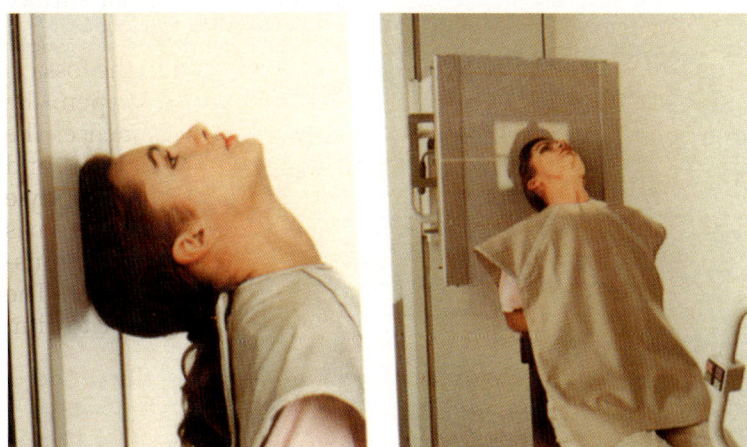

Fig. 4.11: Positioning of the patient in submentovertex projection

Position of the Central X-ray Beam

The central beam is perpendicular to the image receptor, directed from below the mandible towards the vertex of the skull (hence the name Submentovertex or SMV), and centered about 2 cm anterior to a line connecting the right and left condyles.

Resultant Image

The midsagittal plane (represented by an imaginary line extending from the interproximal space of the maxillary central incisor through the nasal septum, to the middle of the anterior arch of the atlas, and to the dens) should divide the skull image in to symmetric halves.

The buccal and lingual cortical plates of mandible should be projected as uniform oblique lines.

An underexposed view is required for the evaluation of the zygomatic arches.

Reverse Towne's Projection

This projection shows the condylar heads and necks.

Indications

1. High fractures of condylar necks.
2. Intracapsular fractures of TMJ.
3. Investigation of the quality of the articular surfaces of the condylar heads in TMJ disorders.
4. Condylar hypoplasia or hyperplasia.

Image Receptor and Patient Placement

1. The image receptor is placed in front of the patient, perpendicular to the midsagittal and parallel to the coronal plane.
2. The patients head is tilted downward so that the canthomeatal line forms a 25- to 30-degree angle with the image receptor.
3. To improve the visualization of the condyles, the patient's mouth is open so that the condylar heads are located inferior to the articular eminence.
4. When requesting this image to evaluate the condyles, it is necessary to specify "Open mouth, reverse-towne" otherwise a standard towne view of the occiput may result.

Position of the Central X-ray beam

The central beam is perpendicular to the image receptor and parallel to patient's midsagittal planes and is centered at the level of the condyles (Fig. 4.12).

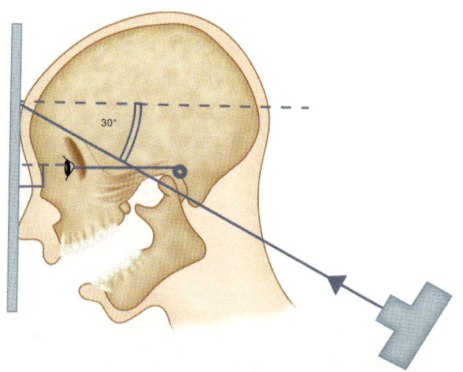

Fig. 4.12: Projection of the central ray

Resultant Image

1. The midsagittal should divide the skull image into two symmetric halves.
2. The petrous ridge of the temporal bone should be superimposed at the inferior part of the occipital bone and the condylar heads should be projected inferior to the articular eminence.

OTHER PROJECTIONS

Cephalometric Projections

The lateral skull and the Posteroanterior Caldwell projection are classic views of the skull. They are used chiefly by orthodontists for assessing and measuring variations in cranial form. These projections are inadequate for details of the temporomandibular joint. The lateral skull projection superimposes the joint structures, obscuring all but gross form and symmetry. PA projection obscures the mandibular condylar processes within the shadows of the temporal bones, because the condyle lies between the mastoid process and the articular eminence.

Xeroradiography

Xeroradiography provides finer and clearer images of the temporomandibular joint because of the wide latitude and edge enhancement inherent characteristic of this modality. A serious drawback of this technique is the unavoidable higher dose of radiation at the skin surface. This dose may be up to 2.4 to 16.2 times higher than with conventional techniques. Therefore, xeroradiography is not a practical method.

BIBLIOGRAPHY

1. Aquilino SA, Matteson SR, Holland GA, Phillips C. Evaluation of condylar position from temporomandibular joint radiographs. J Prosthet Dent 1985;53(1): 88–96.
2. Christiansen EL, Thompson JR. A book on Temporomandibular Joint Imaging. St.Lovie 1990 Mosby,pp39–53.
3. D Carl Dixon, Gar S Graham, Robert B Mayhew, Larrey J Oesterle, David Simms, Wayne P Pierson. The validity of transcranial radiography in diagnosing TMJ anterior disc displacement: JADA 1984;108;615–18.

4. Eric Whaite's Essentials of Dental Radiography and Radiology. Third edition, pp. 371–9.
5. Guidelines for Diagnosis and Management of Disorders Involving the TMJ and Related Musculoskeletal Structures approved by American Society of Temporomandibular Joint Surgeons II.
6. Mongini F. The importance of radiography in the diagnosis of TMJ dysfunctions: a comparative evaluation of transcranial radiographs and serial tomography. J Prosthet Dent 1981; 45; 2:186–98.
7. Murphy WA Adams RJ, Gilula, Barbier JY. Magnification radiography of the temporomandibular joint: technical consideration. Radiology 1979;133:524.
8. Preti G, Fava C. Lateral transcranial radiography of temporomandibular joints, I. Validity in skulls and patients. J Prosthet Dent 1988,59;1:85–93.
9. Pullinger AG, Hollender L. Assessment of mandibular condyle positions: a comparison of transcranial radiographs and linear tomograms. Oral Surg Oral Med Oral Pathol 1985;60:329–34.
10. Sharon L. Brooks, et al. Imaging of the temporomandibular joint Oral Surg Oral Med Oral Pathol Oral Radiol Endod 1997;83:609–18.
11. White SC and Pharoah MJ. Oral Radiology principles and interpretation, fifth Edition published by Elsevier pp.213-15,538–48.
12. White and Pharaoh. Oral Radiology, Principles and interpretation. 5th Edition,pp. 245–264.

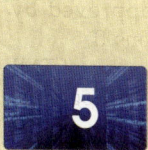

Tomography and Panoramic Imaging

5

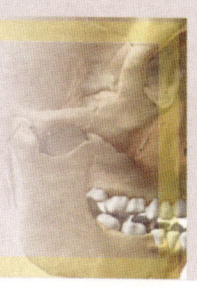

INTRODUCTION

The word tomogram comes from the greek words, *tomos*, a section, and *gramma*, a writing. Tomography, also called body section radiography is a process by which an image of a layer within the body is produced while images of structures above or below that layer are made invisible by blurring. Other terms used are laminagraphy, planigraphy, and zonography (thick section tomography).

Karol Mayer, a radiologist, made the first known attempt at tomography in 1914. Mayer moved the X-ray tube side to side during a chest radiograph, and as a result only the heart was in focus. The predecessor of modern tomographic units was designed in 1921 by Andre-Edmund-Marie Bocage, a French physician. Body section laminagraphy was an established technique by the middle of the 1930s.

Petrilli, a physician, and Gurley, a dentist, were the first investigators of record to make tomograms of the temporomandibular joint in the United States. They experimented with tomograms because they believed that little could be interpreted from TMJ plain films. Rickets was a forerunner in the investigation and use of linear tomography for TMJ disorders. Pantomography was developed in 1960s, chiefly for the purpose of providing broad coverage of the mandibulofacial area in a single image.

APPLICATIONS OF TOMOGRAPHIC METHODS FOR THE TEMPOROMANDIBULAR JOINT

Linear Tomography

In 1930, in an effort to overcome some of the problem enumerated, linear tomography was incorporated as an additional X-ray method.

Linear tomography was found, however, to be too crude a method for evaluating the complex anatomic structures of the head and neck. Thus it has been largely abandoned by the diagnostic radiologist in the study of the TMJ.

Compared to plain films and pantomograms, linear tomograms are able to isolate joint structures without angular distortion, involve only slightly higher absorbed radiation dose, and are better to distinguish fractures than plain films.

The basic tube movement patterns for tomographic blurring in linear tomography are either parallel or perpendicular to the axis of the body. Bony structures oriented perpendicular to the tomographic plane of motion generally are visualized better than those parallel to the plane of motion because of the inherent streaking of linear tomograms. Hyperdense or hypodense areas outside the tomographic plane influence the radiographic density of adjacent structures within the tomographic plane.

The linear streak artefacts caused by adjacent structures of contrasting density can be reduced by:

1. Using a different blurring motion
2. Using a sharper focal plane
3. Changing the radiographic relationships of the body part under study by altering the patient's position.

Pluridirectional Tomography

This is a type of tomography using a pluridirectional medical X-ray unit, designed specifically for modern tomography. This device is employed to study the TMJ. With this unit, it is now possible to detect subtle abnormalities of the condylar articular surface, the joint space, as well as the fossa. Pluridirectional, complex motion tomography was considered the gold standard technique for TMJ imaging in the early 1970s. Most radiologists no longer consider the same because of the invention of newer techniques such as computed tomography and magnetic resonance imaging. As with linear tomography, multiplanar tomographic TMJ images may be made in any suitable diagnostic plane. The most common projections are sagittal and coronal, although oblique projection may help to show joint relationships better, particularly when condylar angles are greater than normal (24 to 25 degrees).

The value of this method has been stressed in a publication from the Mayo Clinic by Stanton and Baker. They state that "soon after routine lateral tomography was begun in July, 1973, overall quality improved greatly and diagnostic detection rate and accuracy increased."

These findings are confirmed by a publication by Rosenberg and Silha. Following points should be stressed concerning the value of pluridirectional tomography in the evaluation of TMJ disorders:

1. It provides a good deal of details about intrinsic bony structures of the condyle, fossa, and surrounding structures.

2. The relationship of the condyle to the fossa may be studied in order to evaluate the joint space. When this is narrowed, it may indicate this disk damage and be the first radiologic sign of an underlying osteoarthritis process.

3. The mobility of the condyle may be evaluated by comparing X-rays taking with the mouth closed, in resting position, with those taken with the mouth open. It is essential to compare the two sides.

4. The presence of suspected tumor and fractures may be ruled out before a final diagnosis is made and treatment instituted.

5. Tomography is extremely valuable for the patient presenting with an atypical clinical picture and for the patient who is not responding to treatment in the usual manner. It is also useful when a prompt relapse takes place during a period of observation.

6. Tomography is especially important for patients who have pain that is not related to occlusal muscle syndrome, but that is likely to be caused by an intrinsic joint disease, such as osteoarthritis or degenerative joint disease.

7. In examination of infants and children, diagnosis of TMJ problems in infants and children should be very carefully evaluated by means of tomography.

8. Tomography is of value in the postoperative period. An operative procedure may cause considerable changes in the TMJ that are difficult to evaluate. Some operative procedures involve the placement of a partial or complete

prosthesis in one or both joints. Following such an operative procedure, a base-line study should be obtained in order to determine the exact location of the prosthesis. If any problems arise in the postoperative period, this information should prove of great value.

9. Tomography may be used in evaluating the efficacy of mandibular occlusal splints.

10. Before planning extensive dental rehabilitation, clinical evaluation of the TMJ is advisable, even if the patient is free of symptoms. In cases of doubt, a tomographic examination is suggested. This may avoid problems at a later date. Latent or subclinical TMJ disease may be activated into a painful problem by extensive dental work.

11. In some patients, tomography may be the only source of needed information.

12. Tomography is also employed to study the changes in the TMJ following treatment.

Corrected or Selected Tomography

Corrected or selected tomography employ to improve the diagnostic quality of the TMJ tomography. This is done because the long axis of the condyle in the horizontal plane usually runs obliquely. The medial pole generally points medially and posteriorly, it is essential to determine the degree of obliquity so that the necessary correction is made prior to the tomography examination.

The objective is to rotate the head so that the long axis of the condyle is either parallel to or at right angle to the film. The obliquity of the two condyles is determined by obtaining a conventional film taken in the full-base or submentovertex projection. Straight lines are then drawn through the middle of the long axes of the two condyles. These lines are projected posteriorly to intersect the midsagittal plane. The resultant angles are measured on the two sides. These angles determine the degree of rotation of the head.

In the lateral projection, the tomographic cuts are thus perpendicular to the long axis. It is important to stress that the degree of obliquity on the two sides may be different. Thus every examination is "tailor-made". When the long axis of the condyle does not run obliquely, rotation of the head is unnecessary. It is essential to examine both sides for comparison.

Also, the examination should be undertaken in both the lateral and frontal projections. The lateral tomographic examination is undertaken in both the mouth closed and mouth open positions. It is advisable to include the entire ramus of the mandible when lateral sets of radiographs are obtained. In the lateral projection with the mouth closed, the condyle is seen to occupy the anterior portion of the cavity of the fossa. The joint space is occupied primarily by the disk, which acts as a cushion or shock absorber, separating the bony structures joint space, superiorly and posteriorly, should measure at least 2.5 mm. If the joint space measures 2 mm or less, narrowing of the joint space results and disk damage should be suspected. The following radiologic features should be carefully observed and the two joints compared

1. Shape of the head (round, flattened, irregular);
2. Surface of the anterior and superior aspects of the head (smooth, irregular, notched);
3. Contour of the cortex (intact, interrupted, condensed);
4. Structure of the medulla;
5. Inclination and length of the ramus of the mandible;
6. Abnormalities of the articular eminence;
7. Mobility of the head in relation to the articular eminence;
8. Depth of the fossa;
9. Position of the head in the fossa;
10. Width of the joint space; and
11. Associated abnormalities (tumor, unilateral hyperplasia or hypoplasia).

Circular Tomography

Pullinger and Holland described the variations in the condyle-fossa relationship according to different methods of evaluation in tomograms. A conventional inferosuperior or submentovertex radiograph is produced by positioning the patient's Frankfort plane parallel to the film and perpendicular to the X-ray beam. This radiograph demonstrates the anterior and posterior surfaces of each condyle. An AP tomogram, using a circular motion with a 10° amplitude and providing a cut 6.5 mm thick, is produced by positing the patient's Frankfort plane in a horizontal plane and condyle perpendicular to the X-ray beam. The superior surface of each condyle is demonstrated in this view. Rosenberg et al reported that maximum tomographic images avoiding geometric distortion can be obtained only when the X-ray beam is either perpendicular to the long axis of the condyle for an AP view or directed along the long axis of the condyle for a true lateral view. The correct direction of the X-rays relative to the condyle will also minimize tomographic shadows. The described method of corrected lateral and anterio-posterior cephalometric tomographic technique has the advantage of accommodating the various skull sizes and shapes as well as producing images that will provide maximum diagnostic information. Hansson and others stated in their clinical experience that osseous changes cannot be evaluated with the same accuracy on a midfield magnet as is possible with high field MRI or with multidirectional conventional tomography. The significance of the osseous changes of the TMJ for treatment decisions is relatively limited for patients with internal derangement.

The main importance of osseous changes is staging, which may also serve as an indicator of the progression of the disease in follow-up. Osseous changes are of greater significance in patients with inflammatory arthritis, in whom the radiographic manifestations of the disease are seen primarily in the bone. Hansson et al compare diagnostic findings of osseous component of the TMJ with use of midfield MRI and multidirectional conventional tomography. Hansson et al described the higher prevalence of osseous changes with complex motion conventional tomography compared with midfield MRI. The difference between the two techniques was most obvious in post-operative images. This result is natural because more osseous changes are to be expected after surgery than in normal volunteers and in patients who have not yet undergone surgery. If osseous changes are of clinical significance, the midfield MRI might have to be supplemented with complex motion conventional tomography or other imaging modalities that is more accurate for osseous disease.

PANORAMIC IMAGING

A special tomography technique that produces a panoramic roentgenograms of curved surfaces are obtained by rotating the X-ray tube and film-screen holder around the patient, who is usually in a sitting position. The film holder, which is much longer than the film, has a protective lead front with a narrow slit. The film is exposed through a narrow slit in its holder. The film moves across the slit as the X-ray tube and film holder rotate around the patient. The resultant roentgenogram is a flattened out image of a curved surface, e.g. the mandible, flattened out on the two-dimensional film. Panoramic radiography term derived from *panorama,* "an unobstructed view of a region in every direction".

Tomography— "an X-ray technique for making radiographs of layers of tissue in depth without the interference of tissue above and below that level". It is a technique for producing a single tomographic image of the facial structures that includes both the maxillary and mandibular dental arches and their supporting structures. This is a curvilinear variant of conventional tomography. It is also based on the principle of the reciprocal movement of an X-ray source and an image receptor around a central point or plane, called the image layer, in which the object of interest located (Figs 5.1 and 5.2).

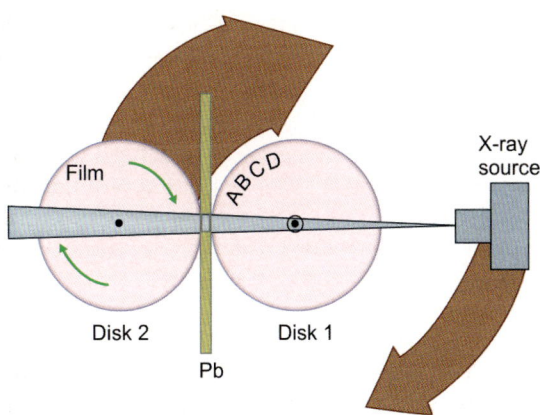

Fig. 5.1: Movement of film and X-ray source about one fixed center of rotation

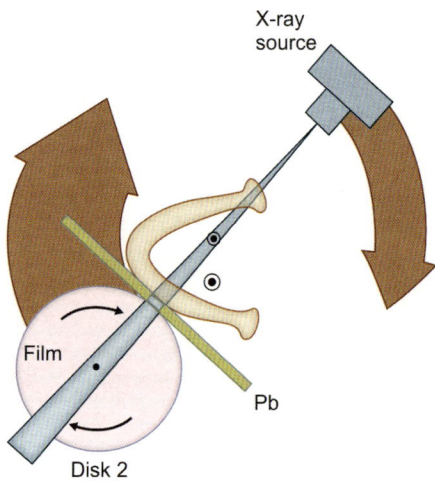

Fig. 5.2: Movement of film and X-ray source about shifting center of rotation

Historical Development

Panoramic radiographs are made using two basically different methods
- The use of an intraoral source of radiation
- The use of extraoral source of radiation

Dr Hisatugu Numata of Japan was 1st to propose (*1933*) and experiment (*1934*) with this method.

In *1946*, Dr.Yrjo Veli Paatero proposed and experimented and demonstrated a slit beam method of panoramic radiography for the dental arches.

Dr. Paatero called this technique pantomography in 1949.

Panoramic radiography is a modified type of tomography or image layer radiography. The patient's dental arch must be positioned within a narrow zone of sharp focus known as the "focal trough"/imaging plane, designed by panoramic machine manufacturers as the ideal patient position to produce the optimum image.

Distortion of the image quality occurs when patients are not properly positioned—such as if the chin is tipped up or down too much, midline rotated off machine center, anterior teeth/jaws too far forward or back. These result in vertical and horizontal magnification and distortion, superimposition of anatomical structures, and some structures being projected out of the field of view. Most panoramic machines offer positioning guides such as lights or plastic guides to position the patient along three major axes: anterior—posterior (too far forward or back), vertically (ala tragus, Frankfort plane, or canthomeatal lines), and midsagittal alignment (patient twisted or rotated).

Teeth and structures lying outside this zone of sharp focus will exhibit blurring, distortion or other artefacts. Therefore, all panoramic machines will have some mechanism for properly positioning the patient's dentition within the focal trough. The trough on older systems can be as narrow as 3 mm in width in the anterior region or as wide as 17 mm on newer panoramic systems, therefore following the manufacturer's guidelines for proper patient positioning is critical in obtaining a quality radiograph. As a general rule, the wider the anterior focal trough the easier it is to position the patient. Proper patient positioning in the focal layer/plane of the panoramic machine is critical for producing successful images. Manufacturers have built into their machines a variety of alignment devices to help ensure the patient positioning process is easy and well visualized by the dental operator. Figures 5.3 and 5.4 show the typical alignment aids provided.

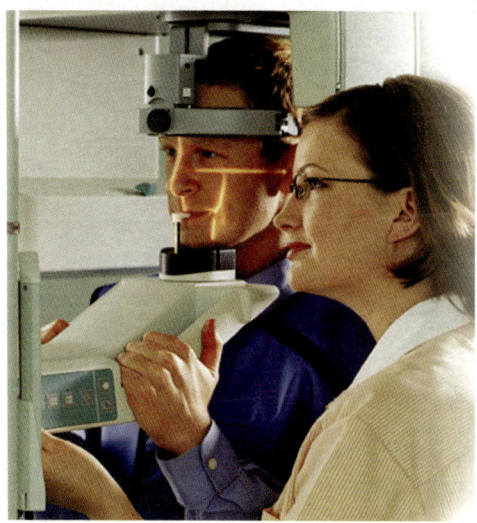

Fig. 5.3: Alignment devices to help ensure the patient positioning

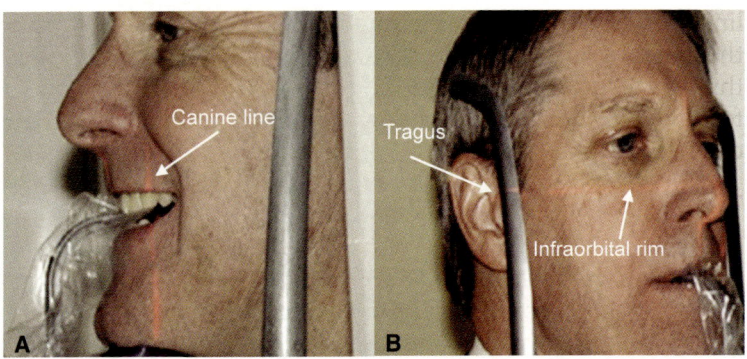

Figs 5.4A and B: Alignment devices to help ensure the patient positioning

The chin rest and the incisal guided bite-block assist positioning the anterior teeth into the smallest region of the focal layer/plane. Lateral/temporal or frontal skull head support bars further assist posterior patient positioning and help to reduce head tilting and horizontal misalignment. Light beam reference lines provide the final visualization for proper patient alignment.

Patient positioning has been shown to be crucial in panoramic imaging of the condyles. If the head is inclined posteriorly, the image of the condyle appears flattened and can simulate the presence of osteophytes. Conversely, if the head is inclined anteriorly, the condyle may appear sclerotic.

Light alignment has three components: mid-sagittal head and skull plane, Frankfort plane, and canine/corner base of nose reference line. The mid-sagittal line is an imaginary plane centred over the midline of the head which divides the anatomy into equal right and left sections when directed between the eyes along the midline of the nose and lips or between the maxillary central incisors, assuming the centrals are present and in an acceptable clinical position. The Frankfort plane line is used to position the patient's head tilt in the vertical plane. The Frankfort plane is an external head reference plane which projects an imaginary line between the superior border of the external auditory meatus or upper portion of the tragus of the ear to the lower infraorbital rim of the eye.

Final forward/backward positioning of the patient's head is determined using the canine/corner base of nose alignment line. This is an imaginary, vertical line that primarily bisects the maxillary canine through the cusp and extends down through a portion of the mandibular canine. The head is moved forward or backward and adjusted until primarily the maxillary canine is bisected with the alignment line.

The Basic Steps

There are several basic steps in taking a panoramic radiograph. These steps will apply to almost any panoramic machine, while some machines have features such as automatic exposure, which reduce the likelihood of exposure error, but do not prevent them entirely. It is important to know the steps and how they affect the outcome of the radiographic process.

When problems occur at any of the steps they will cause unique errors on the resulting radiographs that when recognized, are easy to correct.

1. Set exposure factors, if required.
2. Have patient remove jewellery; place apron on patient's back and shoulders.
3. Have patient bite on bite rod.
4. Adjust the
    a. chin tilt with the Frankfort light.
    b. head rotation with the mid-sagittal light.
    c. forward/backward head position with the canine light.
5. Position the side guides or head support.
6. Have the patient stand up straight.
7. Have patient swallow, place tongue on roof of mouth, and hold still.
8. Take X-ray

Panoramic radiography provides the dentist with an image of the whole dentition and adjacent structures. While panoramic radiography is technique sensitive, by carefully following the ten steps outlined, clear and undistorted radiographs of high diagnostic quality can be consistently obtained.

Updegrave and Philadelphia studied the visualizing the mandibular ramus in panoramic radiography. The structures which exhibit the greatest distortion and indistinctness on the conventionally taken panoramic radiograph are the mandibular rami with their condyloid and coronoid processes.

There are two basic reasons for distorted images of the mandibular ramus on the conventional Panorex radiograph

1. The ramus is positioned outside the focal trough or plane.
2. The ramus is positioned diagonally rather than perpendicularly to the X-ray beam.

The radiographic images of the ascending ramus with its coronoid and condyloid processes can be portrayed more accurately, with minimal distortion, through the use of a modified head position.

Indications

1. As part of orthodontic assessment where there is a clinical need to know the clinical state of the dentition and presence/absence of teeth.
2. To assess bony lesions those are too large to be demonstrated on the intra-oral films.
3. To assess unerupted, impacted, supernumerary teeth.
4. As a part of assessment of periodontal bone support.
5. Assessment of 3rd molars.
6. Assessment of fracture of all part of the mandible, except anterior region.
7. Antral disease particularly to the floor, posterior and medial wall of the antra.
8. Destructive diseases of the articular surface of TMJ.
9. Vertical alveolar height assessment as a part of implant planning.

Principle Advantages

1. Broad coverage.
2. Low patient radiation exposure.
3. Convenience of the examination.
4. Short time procedure.
5. Visual aid in patient education and case presentation.

Disadvantages

1. Do not display the fine anatomic detail available on the Intra-oral periapical films.

2. Not useful in detecting small carious lesions, fine structure of the marginal periodontium, or periapical disease.
3. Proximal surfaces of the premolars overlaps.
4. Unequal magnification and geometric distortion across the image.
5. Cervical spine overlapping over mandibular incisor region.

Panoramic Imaging in Temporomandibular Joint Disorders

The temporomandibular joint (TMJ) remains an elusive structure to examine radiographically, but it is fairly well visualized in panoramic radiographs. The next generation of panoramic machines is programmable, so that better TMJ views are possible. In 1989, panoramic machines with excellent TMJ imaging capability are available.

Condylar Aplasia, Hypoplasia, Hypertrophy, and Hyperplasia

The term "aplasia" means lack of development of a part, and, on rare occasions, condylar aplasia occurs. Hypoplasia means defective or incomplete development of a part. In comparing the right and left condyles, radiographic differences up to 3 mm are considered normal. The proximity of the sigmoid notch to the zygomatic arch may be an indication of condylar hypoplasia.

Hypertrophy means an increase in size of a part due to an increase in size of its constituent cells. The degree of hypertrophy may be relative owing to a projection error caused by unequal magnification of the panoramic image from one side to the other. When this projection error occurs, the ramus on the affected side, but not the body of the mandible, is usually wider.

Hyperplasia means an abnormal increase in the number of cells. According to Worth hyperplasia of the condyles may be divided in to three basic types. In type Ist various attempts at remodelling produce a normally shaped but much larger head of the condyle with a thickened neck area. In type IInd no remodelling takes place, and the head of the condyle is replaced by a globular mass, which may, in some cases, resemble an inverted L. Type IIIrd is probably an exuberant response to the inflammation of degenerative joint disease.

Coronoid Process Enlargement

Coronoid process enlargement is an unusual occurrence but an important consideration in the diagnosis of painless limitation of mandibular opening. The limited opening is caused by impingement of the enlarged coronoid process by the inferior and medial aspects of the malar bone.

Bilateral enlargement is much less frequently encountered and is usually due to idiopathic hyperplasia.

Radiographic Features

When the condition is unilateral, comparison of the affected side with the normal side will reveal an enlarged coronoid process. Additionally, when the enlargement is caused by a neoplasm, the shape of the coronoid process may be altered. When bilateral, the enlargement is usually due to hyperplasia. In this instance, the coronoid processes will appear abnormally large but normal in shape. In cases unilateral or bilateral the standard panoramic view and the special TMJ series provide excellent visualization of the coronoid process.

CONDYLAR ANKYLOSIS

Brief Overview and Radiographic Features

True ankylosis of the TMJ requires bony union between the head of the glenoid fossa.

Zygomaticocoronoid Ankylosis

Zygomaticocoronoid ankylosis is an extremely rare condition, with less than a dozen cases reported in the literature, but it remains an important consideration in the differential diagnosis of progressive painless limitation of mandibular opening.

Radiographic Features

Panoramic films usually show a lack of movement of the coronoid processes when comparing the closed and open views. The submentovertex view may show a close approximation of the coronoid process and the medial aspect of the zygoma. On occasion, mineralization may be discernible between the two bones.

MYOFASCIAL PAIN–DYSFUNCTION SYNDROME (TMJ SYNDROME)
Brief Overview and Radiographic Features

Myofascial pain–dysfunction (MPD) syndrome is now a well-recognized symptom complex that predominantly affects females under the age of 40.

Radiographically, MPD syndrome shows no degenerative alterations of the TMJ in the early stages. There may be a unilateral lack of translation on opening (a radiographic sign of deviation), or there may be lack of concentricity of the head of the condyle in the fossa. MPD syndrome may lead to anterior disk displacement with or without reduction or disk perforation.

DEGENERATIVE JOINT DISEASE
(Osteoarthritis, Hypertrophic Arthritis, Arthritis Deformans)

Degenerative joint disease occurs in about half the population over the age of 50. When the TMJ is involved, the condition is unilateral in about two-thirds of the patients. It is considered part of the aging process but may develop from a single traumatic episode, as a result of long-standing MPD syndrome, or as a sequela to functional disorders of the disk.

Radiographic Features

Radiographically: narrowing of the joint space, with or without painful or nonpainful limitation of mandibular movement; facet formation on the head of the condyle, which may be small or large with a flat or irregular surface; subchondral sclerosis, which is a consideration of reactive dense bone on the surface of the condyle: surface erosions, which may look like cupped-out areas on the articular surface of the condyle or cyst like areas in the medial or lateral aspect known as osteoarthritis or Ely's cyst; osteophytes or spur formation, the latter being the better of the two terms. The spur may be small or large, resembling a hawk beak, and is most frequently seen at the anterior aspect of a facet but may occur anywhere on the head of the condyle. The articular eminence and fossa may exhibit many of the same changes.

Rheumatoid Arthritis (Still's Disease)

Rheumatoid arthritis begins early in life, often in the third decade. In a juvenile form of the disease (Still's disease) arrested mandibular development may result in micrognathia, with a retrognathic "Andy Gump" facial profile. Rheumatoid arthritis tends to involve multiple joints, often bilaterally. In most cases a positive rheumatoid factor is present serologically. The disease may be severe and crippling when not controlled and in the TMJ, partial or complete ankylosis may develop.

Radiographic Features

Rheumatoid arthritis is characterized by osteolysis, and eventually the entire condylar head is lost. Ankylosis and an anterior open bite are frequent sequelae.

TMJ OSTEOMA

Osteomas are benign neoplasms of normal bone occurring on the head and neck of the condyle and the upper portions of the ramus.

CONDYLAR CHONDROMA AND OSTEOCHONDROMA

The chondroma is a rare benign neoplasm of mature cartilage, which sometimes ossifies to some degree, when it may be referred to as osteochondroma. The osteochondroma is the most common of all benign tumors of bone but remains rare in the jaws.

Radiographic Features

The chondroma most certainly begins as radiolucency, as the neoplastic proliferation of cartilage replaces bone. As ossification occurs, opacity in varying degrees may result, with an eventual enlargement of the head of the condyle, resembling an osteoma or hyperplasia.

The high prevalence of minor condylar changes seen in both the TMD and general dental population could reflect positioning artefact, rather than remodelling. In another study, when panoramic radiography was compared with tomography (polytomography or spiral tomography) as the gold standard, specificity was high for the presence or absence of osteophytes

(0.90) and condylar flattening (0.85), while sensitivity was unacceptable (0.29 and 0.33, respectively). This would indicate that when evaluating panoramic images for condylar flattening or presence of osteophytes, false positives are less likely, while false negatives can occur frequently. Currently there is significant controversy regarding the utility of panoramic radiographic imaging in both general practice and when evaluating TMD patients.

Recent articles do not support the use of panoramic radiography in diagnosis of TMD. A recent article in the Journal of the American Dental Association claims a panoramic image should be used when the goal is to identify gross osseous changes in the TMJ. This same article notes that panoramic radiography should not be used for screening of disease in the absence of signs or symptoms of a problem. In a general practice setting, there is support for use of panoramic radiography in patients with pain. Crow et al found a high prevalence of minor condylar changes in both TMD and non-TMD patients. This implies that minor morphological changes in the radiographic image of the condyle in TMD patients may have no relevance and should not be used to infer a diagnosis. This does not imply that panoramic radiography has no place in diagnostic evaluation of the facial pain patient; it clearly has the potential to rule out dental or other diseases that mimic or contribute to facial pain. These findings suggest that panoramic radiography is of no more than limited value in diagnosis of TMD, and minor condylar discrepancies may have no significance in TMD.

Laster et al studied the accuracy of panoramic radiography in detecting mandibular anatomy and asymmetry. This study showed a general lack of sensitivity for subtle asymmetry detection and poor specificity for "mis-positioned" skulls rotated or shifted to a clinically relevant degree.

Epstein et al studied the utility of panoramic imaging of the temporomandibular joint in patients with temporomandibular disorders. Panoramic radiography has frequently been used as a simple, low-cost method to evaluate the bony structures of the TMJ. In this technique the lateral slope and central portions of the TMJ are visualized because of the oblique orientation of the beam with respect to the long axis of the condyle, but the depiction of the articular eminence and fossa is not adequate for diagnosis of other than advanced changes of shape and structure because of the nature of the imaging and superimposition by the base of the skull and zygomatic arch. Although the findings from this consecutive series of 55 patients with facial pain confirm that the panoramic radiograph can show moderate to severe structural abnormality of bone.

Even in a high risk population referred for the diagnosis and management of facial pain and jaw dysfunction, panoramic imaging had little impact on the diagnosis, further investigation, or treatment. This study assessed the utility of panoramic imaging in a series of patients with facial pain and TMD and did not demonstrate the need for use in all patients with such symptoms. Rather, it is recommended that imaging be performed when clinical findings are directly related to the TMJ, particularly in individuals with significant joint findings or lack of response to therapy.

BIBLIOGRAPHY

1. American Dental Association, Council on Dental Materials, Instruments, and Equipment. Panoramic and cephalometric extraoral dental radiograph systems. J Am Dent Assoc 2002;133:1697–98.
2. Arnold Berrett. Radiology of the temporomandibular joint: Symposium on temporomandibular joint dysfunction and treatment; Dent Clin North Am. 1983Jul;27(3):527–40.
3. Chilvarquer I, Freitas A, Glass BJ, Chilvarquer LW, et al. Intercondylar dimension as a positioning factor for panoramic images of the temporomandibular region. Oral Surg Oral Med Oral Pathol 1987;64:768–73.
4. Christiansen EL, Thompson JR. A book on Temporomandibular Joint Imaging. St.Lovie 1990 Mosby. pp. 55–69.
5. Dahlstrom L, Lindvall AM. Assessment of temporomandibular joint disease by panoramic radiography: reliability and validity in relation to tomography. Dentomaxillofac Radiol 1996;25:197–201.
6. Epstein JB, Caldwell J, Black G. The utility of panoramic imaging of the temporomandibular joint in patients with temporomandibular disorders. Oral Surg Oral Med Oral Pathol Oral Radiol Endod 2001; 92:236–9.
7. Hansson LG, Westesson PL, Eriksson L. Comparison of tomography and midfield magnetic resonance imaging for osseous changes of the temporomandibular joint. Oral Surg Oral Med Oral Pathol Endod 1996;82:698–703.

8. HC Crow, E Parks, JH Campbell, DS Stucki, J Daggy. The utility of panoramic radiography in temporomandibular joint assessment. Dentomaxillofacial Radiology 2005;34:91–5.
9. Langland, Langlais; Book on Panoramic Radiology 2nd edition 1989 pp. 415–28.
10. Laster WS, Ludlow JB, Bailey LJ, Hershey HG. Accuracy of measurements of mandibular anatomy and prediction of asymmetry in panoramic radiographic images. Dentomaxillofac Radiol 2005; 34:343–9.
11. Pullinger A, Holland L. Variations in the condyle-fossa relationship according to different methods of evaluation in tomograms. Oral Surg Oral Med Oral Pathol 1986;62:719-27.
12. Reviewed Publication by Dr. Robert A. Danforth Successful Panoramic Radiography pp. 1–15.
13. Rosenberg HM, Richard JG. Temporomandibular articulation tomography: A corrected anteroposterior and lateral cephalometric technique. Oral Surg Oral Med Oral Pathol 1986; 62:198–204.
14. Ruf S, Pancherz H. Is orthopantomography reliable for TMJ diagnosis? An experimental study on a dry skull. J Orofac Pain 1995; 9: 365–74.
15. Rushton VE, Horner K, Worthington HV. Screening panoramic radiology of adults in general dental practice: radiological findings. Br Dent J 2001; 190:495–501.
16. Rushton VE, Horner K, Worthington HV. Routine panoramic radiography of new adult patients in general dental practice: relevance of diagnostic yield to treatment and identification of radiographic selection criteria. Oral Surg Oral Med Oral Pathol Oral Radiol Endod 2002;93:488–95.
17. Thomas Curry, James Dowdey, Robert Murry: Christensen's Physics of Diagnostic Radiology, 3rd edition.
18. Updegrave WJ. Visualizing the mandibular ramus in panoramic radiography. Oral Surg Oral Med Oral Pathol 1971; 31:422–29.
19. White and Pharaoh. Oral Radiology, Principles and interpretation. 5th Edition,pp. 191–209.

Computed Tomography

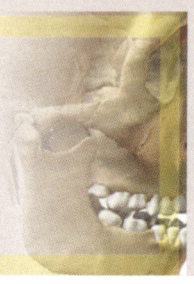

INTRODUCTION

At the Annual Congress of the British Institute of Radiology, in April 1972, Godfrey Hounsfield, a senior research scientist at EMI Limited in Middlesex, England, announced the invention of a revolutionary imaging technique, which he referred to as "computerized axial transverse scanning". The basic concept was quite simple: a thin cross-section of the head, a tomographic slice, was examined from multiple angles with a pencil like narrowly collimated, moving beam of X-rays. A scintillation crystal detected the remnant radiation of this beam, and the resulting analog signal was fed into a computer, digitized, and analyzed by a mathematical algorithm and the data reconstructed as an axial tomographic image. The image produced by this technique is claimed to be 100 times more sensitive than conventional X-ray systems. It demonstrated differences between various soft tissues, never before seen with X-ray imaging techniques.

Since 1972, computed tomography (CT) has had many names: "computerized axial tomography", "computed tomographic scanning", "axial tomography", and "computerized transaxial tomography". Currently the term "computed tomography", abbreviated as CT is most commonly used.

CT scanner consists of a radiographic tube that emits a finely collimated, fan shaped X-ray beam directed to a series of scintillation detectors or ionization chambers. Depending on the scanner's geometry, both the radiographic tube and detectors may rotate synchronously about the patient; or the detectors may form a continuous ring about the patient and the X-ray tube may move in a circle within the detector ring. CT scanners that employ this type of movement for image acquisition are called incremental scanners because the final image set consists of a series of continuous or overlapping axial images (Figs 6.1A and B).

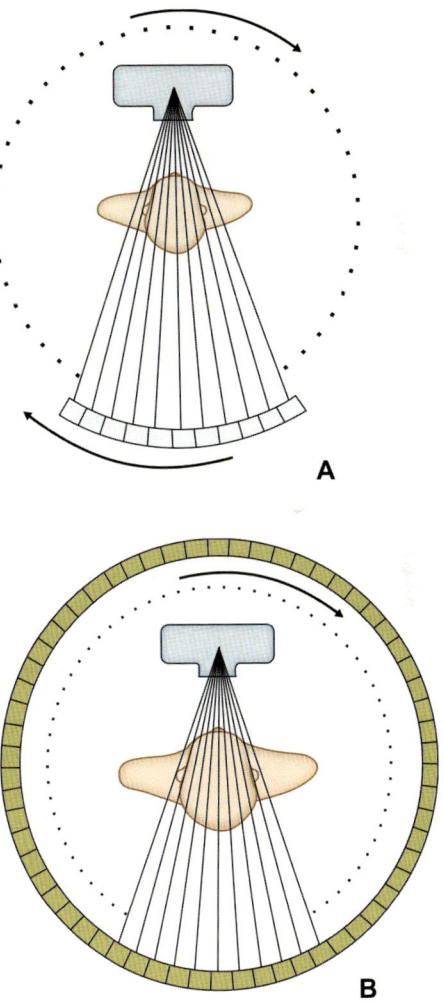

Figs 6.1A and B: Mechanical geometry of CT scanner. (A) both the X-ray tube and the detector array revolve around the patient. (B) only the X-ray tube rotates; radiation detection is accomplished by the use of a fixed circular array of as many as 1000 detectors

The CT image is a digital image, reconstructed by computer, which mathematically manipulates the transmission data obtained from multiple projections. The CT image is recorded and displayed as a matrix of individual blocks called voxels (volume elements). Each square of the image matrix is a pixel. Whereas the size of the pixel (about 0.1 mm) is determined partly by the width of the X-ray beam, which in turn is controlled by the prepatient and postpatient collimators. Voxel length is analogous to the tomographic layer in film tomography (Figs 6.2A to E)

For image display each pixel is assigned a CT number representing density. This number is proportional to the degree to which the material within the voxel has attenuated the X-ray beam. It represents the absorption characteristics, or linear attenuation coefficient, of that particular volume of tissue in the patient. CT numbers, also known as Hounsfield units, may range from –1000 to + 1000, each constituting a different level of optical density. This scale of relative densities is based on air (–1000), water (0), and dense bone (+1000).

Advantages

1. CT completely eliminates the superimposition of images of structures outside the area of interest.
2. Because of inherent high contrast resolution of CT, differences between tissues that differ in physical density by less than 1% can be distinguished. Whereas conventional radiography requires 10% difference in physical density to distinguish between tissues.

Data from single CT imaging procedure consisting of either multiple contiguous or one helical scan can be viewed as images in either axial, coronal, or sagittal planes, depending on the diagnostic task. This is referred to as multiplanar reformatted imaging.

Disadvantages

- CT does involve exposure to radiation in the form of X-rays, but the benefit of an accurate diagnosis far outweighs the risk. The effective radiation dose from this procedure is about 10 mSv, which is about the same as the average person receives from background radiation in three years.

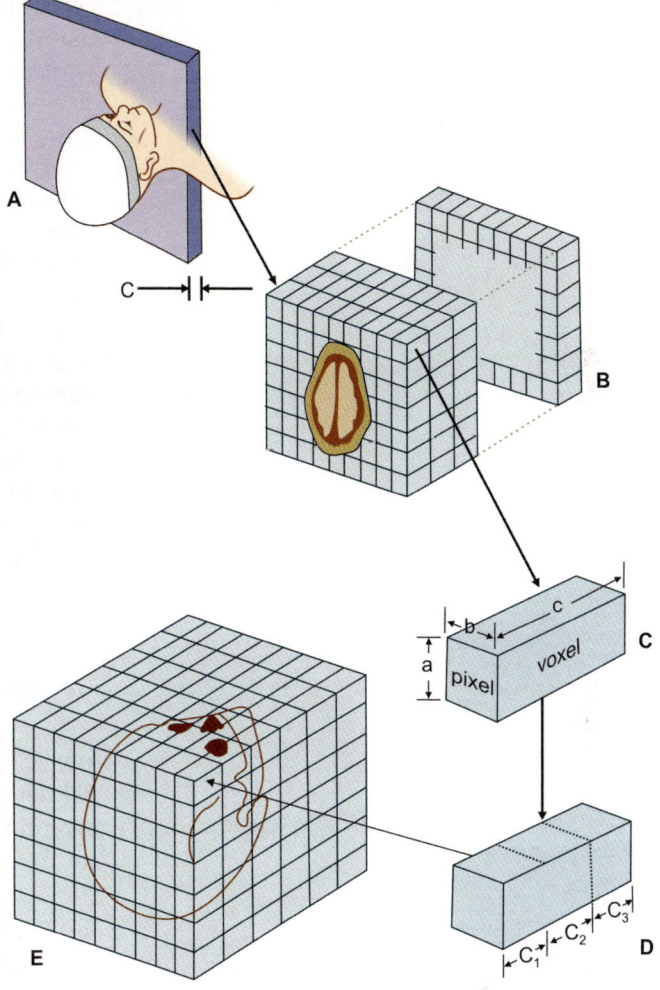

Figs 6.2A to E: CT image formation

- Women should always inform their doctor or X-ray technologist if there is any possibility that they are pregnant.
- Nursing mothers should wait 24 hours after contrast injection before resuming breast feeding.

- There is a risk of serious allergic reaction to iodine-containing contrast material, although very rare but the radiology departments must be well equipped to deal with them.
- A limitation of conventional CT is that although it has a high degree of accuracy within individual slices, but it has relatively low between slice accuracy even with relatively narrow collimation (2 mm) and no interslice gaps.

Recently, CT scanners have been developed that acquire image data in a spiral or helical fashion. With these scanners, while the gantry containing the X-ray tube and detectors revolves around the patient, the table on which the patient is placed continuously advances through the gantry. This results in acquisition of a continuous spiral of data as the X-ray beam moves down the patient.

Because of its high-contrast resolution and ability to demonstrate small differences in soft tissue density, CT has become useful for the diagnosis of the disease in the maxillofacial complex, including the salivary gland and TMJ, However, with the advent of magnetic resonance imaging which has proved superior to CT for depicting soft tissue, the use of CT scanning for assessment of internal derangements of TMJ has decreased significantly.

CT OF TEMPOROMANDIBULAR JOINT

CT of temporomandibular joints is currently the best method for assessing bony pathologic conditions. It is difficult to position a patient within the gantry for true sagittal cuts, and reconstructed sagittal views can be less than ideal. On a sagittal CT scan of a normal joint, the meniscus is located between the condylar head and the articulating surface of the temporal bone. The small soft tissue density anterior and posterior to the point of the articulation between the condyle and the temporal bone represents the anterior and posterior parts of the meniscus. On a CT scan with the condyle open, the meniscus again is located in the normal position. The small amount of tissue anterior and posterior to the point of articulation indicates that the meniscus has maintained a normal position on the condyle.

James Manzione et al reported direct sagittal scanning of the TMJ with the patient lying supine on a stretcher placed lateral to the gantry and perpendicular to the scanner trolley. The patient's head was then positioned facing up in the gantry in a lateral orientation (Fig. 6.3). The temporomandibular joint was scanned from lateral to medial using contiguous 2 mm thick sections, in both open and closed mouth positions. He concluded that direct sagittal CT scanning of the temporo-mandibular joint has the potential for providing a non-invasive evaluation of the meniscus as well as bony abnormalities of the articulating surfaces.

Axial and coronal views are excellent for assessing normal and abnormal osseous anatomy. CT images are rarely used as the primary mode of diagnosing disc displacement. In most instances, accurate differentiation between meniscal tissue and portions of the lateral pterygoid muscle is difficult on CT. Disc displacement is frequently inferred from the degenerative changes seen on CT scan images, such as flattening of the anterior superior slope of the condyle, increased sclerosis, gross remodelling of the condylar head and articular eminence, and osteophyte formation. 3-D CT can be useful in cases of gross asymmetry for planning orthognathic surgery or joint reconstruction. TMJ computed tomography gained popularity between 1982 and 1985. It was introduced in the United States by Suarez and coworkers in 1980. Clinical studies that evaluated CT against pluridirectional tomography, arthrography and surgery initially appeared favorable for CT.

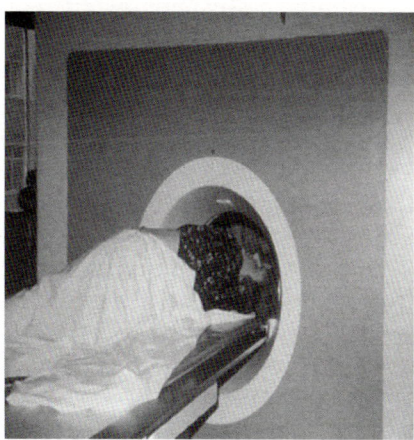

Fig. 6.3: Positioning of the patient for CT of the temporomandibular joint

APPLICATIONS OF CT IN TMJ

1. CT is not indicated for routine radiographic examination of the temporomandibular joint. But it is ideal for craniofacial trauma, being superior to plain film radiography or even tomography.
2. CT is mainly indicated in craniofacial pain of suspicious origin.
3. Tumors in the infratemporal fossa, parapharyngeal spaces, and periarticular tissues are best detected with CT.
4. It is the best method for delineating the details of osteoarthritis.
5. CT is also useful for imaging malpositioned TMJ disc, however sometimes the tendinous attachment of the lateral pterygoid muscle can be mistaken for the articular disc, particularly on the highlighted section.

For best understanding and diagnosing of pathology, simultaneous viewing of both the joints is important for comparison of morphology of symptomatic and asymptomatic joints. This is best accomplished in the true axial plane of head (parallel to the Reid's base line). Axial plane, thin section scanning is ideal for depicting two dimensional TMJ structure and the relationships of the hard and soft tissues because it provides superior coverage of the head and face, is more comfortable for the patient than direct sagittal scanning, and yields a data matrix more easily and quickly manipulated than that obtained by coronal and sagittal scanning.

If scanning is restricted to the coronal and sagittal without vertical reformatting, it is likely that important anatomic features and relationships will be overlooked. For example, the contours of the glenoid fossa and the articular eminence reciprocate the morphology of the condyle and often provide the indirect information on the disc position. CT has an advantage that the data can be manipulated, that is, the images can be viewed in anatomic planes other than the planes of acquisition. Serial axial plane images can be vertically reformatted to paraxial images in any vertical plane.

Edwin Christiansen et al used CT to make computer assisted measurements of the joint space surrounding the condyle in patients and to correlate joint space data with positions of the articular disc. Edwin Christiansen et al, studied the computed tomograms of temporomandibular joints in 25 patients were retrospectively evaluated for condylar position and joint space with general electric computer software.

Computed tomography scans of the TMJ were made in the axial plane with the teeth in centric occlusion and measurements were made from vertically reformatted images. Inter-articular joint spaces were measured anterosuperiorly, superiorly, posterosuperiorly, and posteriorly from the condylar surfaces. They conclude:

1. If the disk is normally located on the condyle, the anterosuperior joint space is consistent across the condyle.
2. If the disk is medial to the condyle, the superior joint space widens.
3. In only those joints in which the disk lay anteromedial to the condyle did absence (0.20 mm) of joint space occur.
4. If the disk is normal, anterolateral, or medial, the anterosuperior joint space appears essentially the same.
5. Absence of joint space occurs most frequently in the lateral two-thirds of the condyle.
6. Joint space narrowing can be focal in its location.
7. Differences in joints space between male and female patients were noted, although the significance of these differences is unclear.

3-D CT

Multiplanar CT imaging has made a significant contribution to diagnosis. However, these images are two dimensional and require a certain degree of mental integration by the viewer for interpretation; this limitation has led to the development of computer programme that reformat data acquired from axial CT scans in to three dimensional images (3-D CT).

DATA ACQUISITION

In CT scan of maxillofacial region, a high resolution power is needed because the area of interest is specific. Spiral/helical CT scanners generate adequate image data to produce three dimensional images with less scanning time and less patient radiation exposure as compared to conventional CT scans.

These newer machines feature a continuous scanner rotation and object transport (tabletop movement). Although the high resolution data generated from spiral/helical CT scanners is preferred for three dimensional imaging, three-dimensional images can also be generated by conventional (nonspiral) CT scanners when adequate scanning parameters are selected. The authors examine the jaws using the data obtained with a tabletop feed speed of 1 to 3 mm per rotation. This technique produces volume image data that are reconstructed to continuous slice CT images with a slice thickness of 1 to 3 mm and with the slices overlapping one another. This overlapping increases the quality of these 3-D CT images.

IMAGE RENDERING SYSTEMS

3-D CT images must be rendered in a computer. Most current spiral/helical CT scanners are supplied with optional three-dimensional rendering software. The three-dimensional rendering software occupies a lot of space in the computer interface of the CT scanner. This need for memory space may interfere with the CT examination of the next patient. A practical alternative is to use an independent work station or personal computer. In three-dimensional imaging a high speed computer is needed. When PCs are used the clinician needs to transfer the CT image data from the CT scanner to the independent computer system via the computer network or on a variety of data storage disc. The development of diagnostic image data format standards, such as the digital imaging and communication in medicine (DICOM) standard, improves the possibility of using independent computers for 3-D CT imaging.

IMAGING TECHNIQUE

The authors describe some of the most currently available 3-D CT imaging techniques as they may be applied to the maxillofacial region. This 3-D CT imaging technique can be divided into the following groups.
1. Multiplanar reformatting (MPR) and dental MPR
2. Shaded surface display (SSD)
3. Volume rendering
4. Maximum intensity projection (MIP)
5. Model production and virtual reality.

MULTIPLANAR REFORMATTING AND DENTAL MULTIPLANAR REFORMATTING

Glenn et al proposed the MPR technique in 1975. MPR displays CT slices in any direction in orthogonal as well as in curvilinear planes, e.g. reconstructed coronal and sagittal MPR images show the relationship between the root apices and the maxillary sinus without an additional coronal or sagittal scan.

The MPR technique has other dental implications as well, such as software designed for preoperative implant treatment planning, like dentascan, evaluated by many clinicians.

Preda et al used MPR to evaluate the localization of impacted maxillary canines. Abrahams and Glassberg investigated an association of focal maxillary sinus disease with periodontal disease using maxillary dental MPR images.

Bordner and Bar-ziv investigated the characteristics of new bone formation after marsupialization of jaw cysts.

SHADED SURFACE DISPLAY

Shaded surface display is useful if there is a need to look at the surface of a structure, such as bone, teeth, or skin, in a three dimensional image. Herman and Liu developed one of these earlier imaging techniques.

To visualize the selected structure, its threshold value must be defined. This thresholding process separates the soft tissue and bone by defining a specific range of Hounsfield units (HU), or CT number. Because an SSD image consists of millions of thresholded three-dimensional matrices of volume elements (voxels), this differentiation makes it possible to separate the surface of the skin or of a bone in a 3-D CT image. Bony structures of the skull or jaws or soft tissue of the skin can be looked at by changing the HU threshold. To see the skin surface a minimum threshold of less than −300 HU is selected. To look at the surface of bone, a minimum threshold of 150 to 200 HU is entered. If a minimum threshold of more than 1000 HU is selected, the roots of teeth are usually represented in the three-dimensional image because the alveolar bone has a lower HU than dentin.

One major advantage of SSD is its faster speed. This speed allows the clinician to reposition interactively and manipulate three-dimensional images rapidly. Therefore, it is beneficial in the diagnosis and treatment of many dental problems such as jaw fractures, maxillofacial deformities and tumors. Takashi et al studied coronoid hyperplasia using 3-D CT.

Naito et al measured alveolar bone levels with 3-D CT images and revealed that 3-D CT may yield precise assessment of bone defects caused by periodontal disease.

VOLUME RENDERING

Shimizu et al reported that although SSD provides excellent image quality with three dimensional displays, the selection of a single threshold and transparency of 0% results in less information. Also voxels with a CT value below the chosen threshold are not displayed in the 3-D CT image. Shimizu et al proposed a type of SSD in which multiple thresholds and transparencies are selected. If the number of thresholds is increased to a sufficient level, the resultant image is a volume-rendered three-dimensional image. The advantage of volume rendering is that the clinician can see the inner features of a three-dimensional structure in such an image.

The high flexibility of volume rendering allows a further modification of 3-D CT imaging techniques. Even 3-D CT images resembling conventional panoramic radiographs and cephalograms can be created. These images can be used as substitutes for radiographs because the fundamental source of the imaging in both CT and radiography is the same.

Lee et al demonstrated the utility of volume-rendering 3-D CT in the head and neck region. Using volume-rendering CT, the authors looked at post-surgical displacement of hard tissue structures, such as temporomandibular joint and hyoid bone, post-surgical changes in the soft tissue structures, such as the muscles of mastication and salivary glands, and post-surgical changes in the pharyngeal airway in mandibular prognathism patients treated with mandibular setback osteotomy.

MAXIMUM INTENSITY PROJECTION

MIP is used to create angiographic images from CT and MR imaging data. In this technique, the intensity of each voxel in the resulting image is the maximum intensity encountered along a line from the viewer's eye as it traverses the volume.

Sawamura et al in the performed 3-D CT angiographic imaging using MIP and SSD techniques in the maxillofacial region, including a facial arteriovenous malformations.

MODEL PRODUCTION AND VIRTUAL REALITY THREE-DIMENSIONAL IMAGING

Several methods have been proposed to produce life sized three-dimensional models that are based on CT data. Milling methods to produce the model use hardened polyurethane, wax, or other materials.

The primary advantage of model production is for preoperative surgical planning, requiring a life-sized model of the patient's skull. These models can be useful for educational purposes. Kishi et al created resin skull models with hyperplasia of the mandibular condyle and fractures of the maxilla and mandible and coronoid process.

Lill et al discussed the accuracy of measurements obtained from a hardened polyurethane skull model and reported that the surgeons using this technique should consider the possible discrepancies between the model and real skull when making preoperative assessments.

A further disadvantage of this technique may be the expense in creating the model. In dentistry this technique can be used to observe the interior of the maxillary sinus, salivary ducts, temporomandibular joint space, and root canals. Three-dimensionally reformatting requires that each original voxel, shaped as a rectangular parallel piped or rectangular solid, be dimentionally altered into multiple cuboidal voxels. This process is called interpolation, and it creates sets of evenly spaced cuboidal voxels (cuberilles) that occupy the same volume as the original voxel. The CT numbers of the cuberilles represent the average of the original voxel CT numbers surrounding each of the new voxels. Creation of these new cuboidal voxels allows the image to be reconstructed in any plane without loss of resolution by locating their position in space relative to one another. In construction of the 3-D CT image, only cuberilles representing the surface of the object scanned are projected onto the viewing monitor. The surface formed by these cuberilles may then appear as if illuminated by a light source located behind the viewer. In this manner the visible surface of each pixel is assigned a gray level value, depending on its distance from and orientation to the light source. Once constructed, 3-D CT images may be further manipulated by rotation about any axis to display the structure imaged from many angles. Also external surfaces of the image can be removed electronically to reveal concealed deeper anatomy.

Ciccarelli R et al examined 347 patients with TMJ disorders using two different 3rd generation CT units. They concluded that CT with 3-D reconstructions as the gold standard technique for functional TMJ studies. Even though it provides no information on the joint disk—which MRI does—3-D CT permits easy and accurate measurements of both TMJ sides which can support clinical finding.

BIBLIOGRAPHY

1. Akitoshi K, Yoshiko A, Robert P. Langlais. Three Dimensional Computed Tomography Imaging in Dentistry. Dental Clinics of North America 2000;44 (2):395–410.
2. Bordner L, Bar-Ziv J. Characteristics of bone formation following marsupialisation of jaw cysts. Dentomaxillofac Radiol 1998;27:166–71.
3. Christiansen EL, Thompson JR. A book on Temporomandibular Joint Imaging. St.Lovie 1990 Mosby. pp.92–8.
4. Ciccarelli R, Di Salle F, Guidi G, Lavorgna G, Sagliocco R, Rotondo A, Smaltino F. Three-dimensional imaging with computerized tomography. Etiologic considerations and methods for studying temporomandibular joints. Radiol Med (Torino). 1998 May; 95(5): 417–23.
5. Edwin L Christiansen, Joseph R. Thompson, Grenith Zimmermen, David Roberts, Anton N. Hasso, David B. Hinshaw, Sigvard Kopp, Loma Linda, Malmo: Computed tomography of condylar and articular disc positions within the temporomandibular joint. Oral Surg Oral Med Oral Pathol 1987;64:757–67.
6. Kishi K, Hasegawa I, Shigehara H, et al. Clinical application of 3- D C T and 3-D plastic model in the maxillo – facial region. Oral Radiol 13: 83–92, 1997.
7. Lill W, Solar P, Ulm G, et al. Reproducibility of 3-dimensional CT – assisted model production in the maxillofacial area. Br. J Oral Maxillofac Surg 1992,30:232–36.
8. N Guler, S Uckan, P Imirzalioglu, S Acikgozoglu. Temporomandibular joint internal derangement: Relationship between joint pain and MR

grading of effusion and total protein concentration in the joint fluid. Dentomaxillofac Radiol 2005;34:175–81.

9. Preda L, Fianza AL, Maggio EMD, et al. The use of spiral computed tomography in the localization of impacted maxillary canines. Dentomaxillofac Radiol 1997;26:236–41.

10. Sartoris DJ, Neumann CH, Riley RW. The temporomandibular joint: true saggital computed tomography with meniscus visualization. Radiology 1984;150:250–54.

11. Shimizu T, Yoshikawa S, Uesugi Y et al. Three-dimensional computed tomographic angiography of pulmonary vessels. Radiat Med. 1999,17:151–4.

12. Thomas Curry, James Dowdey, Robert Murry. Christensen's Physics of Diagnostic Radiology. 3rd edition, p. 320.

13. White, Pharaoh. Oral Radiology, Principles and interpretation. 5th Edition,pp 245–64.

14. William C. Scarfe, Allan G. Farman, Predag Sukovic. Clinical Applications of Cone-Beam Computed Tomography in Dental Practice J Can Dent Assoc 2006;72 (1):75–80.

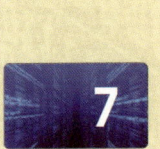

Cone-Beam Computed Tomography

Cone-beam computed tomography (CBCT) systems have been designed for imaging hard tissues of the maxillofacial region. CBCT is capable of providing sub-millimetre resolution in images of high diagnostic quality, with short scanning times (10–70 seconds) and radiation dosages reportedly up to 15 times lower than those of conventional CT scans. CBCT allows the creation in "real time" of images not only in the axial plane but also 2-dimensional (2-D) images in the coronal, sagittal and even oblique or curved image planes—a process referred to as multiplanar reformation (MPR). In addition, CBCT data are amenable to reformation in a volume, rather than a slice, providing 3-dimensional (3-D) information (Fig. 7.1).

TYPES OF CT SCANNERS

Computed tomography can be divided into 2 categories based on acquisition X-ray beam geometry; namely: fan-beam and cone-beam (Fig. 7.2). In fan-beam scanners, an X-ray source and solid-state detector are mounted on a rotating gantry. (Fig. 7.2A). Data are acquired using a narrow fan-shaped X-ray beam transmitted through the patient. The patient is imaged slice-by slice, usually in the axial plane, and interpretation of the images is achieved by stacking the slices to obtain multiple 2-D representations. The linear array of detector elements used in conventional helical fan-beam CT scanners is actually a multi-detector array. This configuration allows multidetector CT (MDCT) scanners to acquire up to 64 slices simultaneously, considerably reducing the scanning time compared with single-slice systems and allowing generation of 3-D images at substantially lower doses of radiation than single detector fan-beam CT arrays.

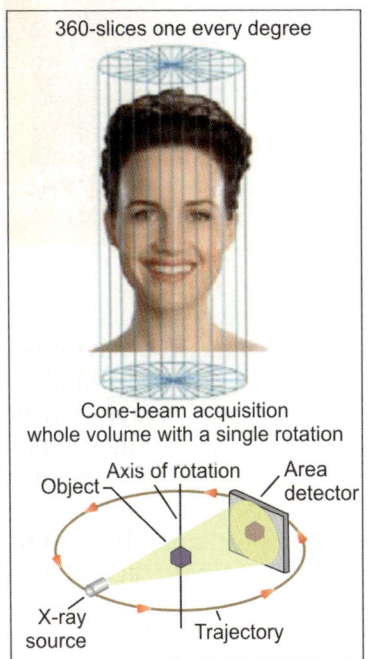
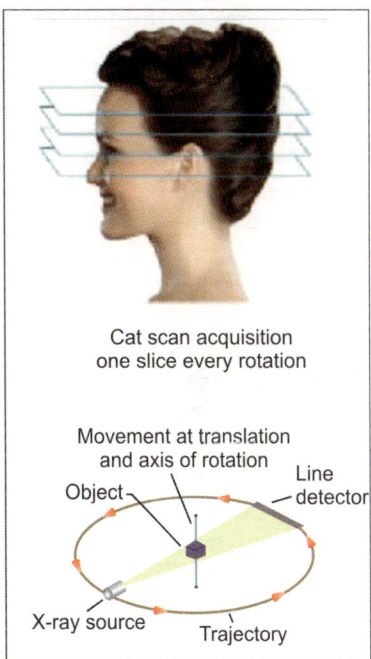

360-slices one every degree

Cone-beam acquisition
whole volume with a single rotation

Object — Axis of rotation   Area detector

X-ray source   Trajectory

Cat scan acquisition
one slice every rotation

Movement at translation
and axis of rotation   Line detector

Object

X-ray source   Trajectory

Fig. 7.1: Differences in image acquisition between cone-beam volume tomography and traditional computed tomography (CT)

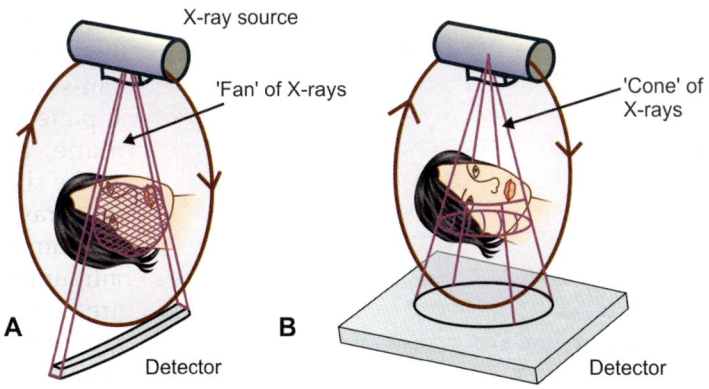

Figs 7.2A and B: X-ray beam projection scheme comparing a single detector array fan-beam CT (A) and cone-beam CT (B) geometry

Cone-Beam CT Technology

CBCT scanners are based on volumetric tomography, using a 2-D extended digital array providing an area detector. This is combined with a 3-D X-ray beam (Fig. 7.2B). The cone-beam technique involves a single 360° scan in which the X-ray source and a reciprocating area detector synchronously move around the patient's head, which is stabilized with a head holder. At certain degree intervals, single projection images, known as "basis" images, are acquired. These are similar to lateral cephalometric radiographic images, each slightly offset from one another. This series of basis projection images is referred to as the projection data. Software programs incorporating sophisticated algorithms including back-filtered projection are applied to these image data to generate a 3-D volumetric data set, which can be used to provide primary reconstruction images in 3 orthogonal planes (axial, sagittal and coronal). Most CBCT units for maxillofacial applications use an image intensifier tube (IIT)–charge coupled device. Recently a system employing a flat panel imager (FPI) was released (i-CAT). The FPI consists of a cesium iodide scintillator applied to a thin film transistor made of amorphous silicon. Images produced with an IIT generally result in more noise than images from an FPI and also need to be pre-processed to reduce geometric distortions inherent in the detector configuration.

Advantages of CBCT

CBCT is well suited for imaging the craniofacial area. It provides clear images of highly contrasted structures and is extremely useful for evaluating bone. The use of CBCT technology in clinical practice provides a number of potential advantages for maxillofacial imaging compared with conventional CT—

- *X-ray beam limitation:* Reducing the size of the irradiated area by collimation of the primary X-ray beam to the area of interest minimizes the radiation dose. Most CBCT units can be adjusted to scan small regions for specific diagnostic tasks. Others are capable of scanning the entire craniofacial complex when necessary.
- *Image accuracy:* The volumetric data set comprises a 3-D block of smaller cuboid structures, known as voxels, each

representing a specific degree of X-ray absorption. The size of these voxels determines the resolution of the image. In conventional CT, the voxels are anisotropic—rectangular cubes where the longest dimension of the voxel is the axial slice thickness and is determined by slice pitch, a function of gantry motion. Although CT voxel surfaces can be as small as 0.625 mm square, their depth is usually in the order of 1–2 mm. All CBCT units provide voxel resolutions that are isotropic—equal in all 3-dimensions. This produces sub-millimetre resolution (often exceeding the highest grade multi-slice CT) ranging from 0.4 mm to as low as 0.125 mm.

- *Rapid scan time:* Because CBCT acquires all basis images in a single rotation, scan time is rapid (10–70 seconds) and comparable with that of medical spiral MDCT systems. Although faster scanning time usually means fewer basis images from which to reconstruct the volumetric data set, motion artifacts due to subject movement are reduced.

- *Dose reduction:* Published reports indicate that the effective dose of radiation (average range 36.9–50.3 microsievert [μSv]) is significantly reduced by up to 98% compared with "conventional" fan-beam CT systems (average range for mandible 1,320–3,324 μSv; average range for maxilla 1,031–1,420 μSv). This reduces the effective patient dose to approximately that of a film-based periapical survey of the dentition (13–100 μSv)18–20 or 4–15 times that of a single panoramic radiograph (2.9–11 μSv).

- *Display modes unique to maxillofacial imaging:* Access and interaction with medical CT data are not possible as workstations are required. Although such data can be "converted" and imported into proprietary programs for use on personal computers, this process is expensive and requires an intermediary stage that can extend the diagnostic phase. Reconstruction of CBCT data is performed natively by a personal computer. In addition, software can be made available to the user, not just the radiologist, either via direct purchase or innovative "per use" licence from various vendors (e.g. Imaging Sciences

International). This provides the clinician with the opportunity to use chair-side image display, real-time analysis and MPR modes that are task specific. Because the CBCT volumetric data set is isotropic, the entire volume can be reoriented so that the patient's anatomic features are realigned. In addition, cursor-driven measurement algorithms allow the clinician to do real-time dimensional assessment.

- *Reduced image artefact:* With manufacturers' artefact suppression algorithms and increasing number of projections, CBCT images can result in a low level of metal artefact, particularly in secondary reconstructions designed for viewing the teeth and jaws.

Application of CBCT Imaging to Clinical Dental Practice

1. Pre-surgical evaluation for implant placement
2. Surgical assessment of pathology
3. TMJ assessment
4. Pre and postoperative assessment of craniofacial fractures
5. In orthodontics to assess the growth and development.

There are different real-time advanced image display techniques, easily derived from the volumetric data set available, explained as under

- *Oblique planar reformation:* This technique creates nonaxial 2-D images by transecting a set or "stack" of axial images. This mode is particularly useful for evaluating specific structures (e.g. TMJ, impacted third molars) as certain features may not be readily apparent on perpendicular MPR images (Fig. 7.3).

- *Curved planar reformation:* This is a type of MPR accomplished by aligning the long axis of the imaging plane with a specific anatomic structure. This mode is useful in displaying the dental arch, providing familiar panorama like thin-slice images (Fig. 7.4A). Images are undistorted so that measurements and angulations made from them have minimal error.

- *Serial transplanar reformation:* This technique produces a series of stacked sequential cross-sectional images orthogonal to the oblique or curved planar reformation. Images are usually thin slices (e.g. 1 mm thick) of known

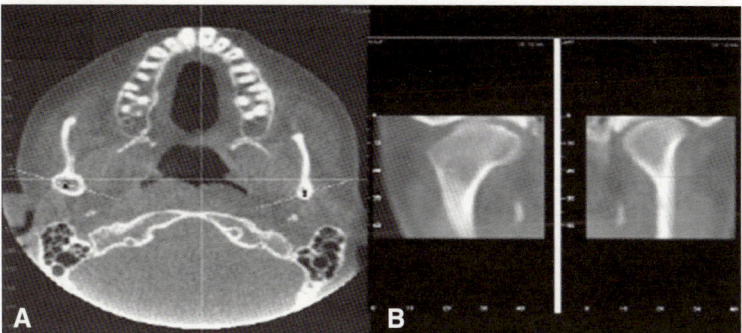

Figs 7.3A and B: Bilateral linear oblique multiplanner reformation through lateral and medial poles of mandibular condyles on axial image (A) and providing corrected coronal, limited field of view, thin-slice temporomandibular views (B) demonstrating right condylar hyperplasia

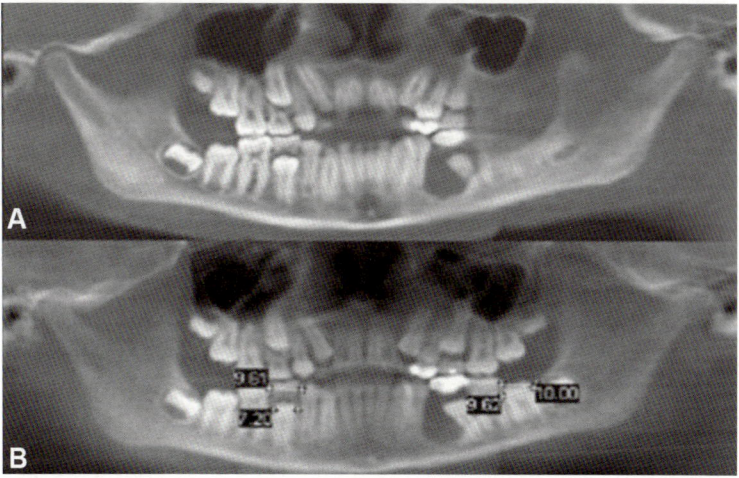

Figs 7.4A and B: Narrow (5.3 mm)(A) and wide (25.6 mm)(B) slice simulated panoramic images providing anatomically accurate measurements

separation (e.g. 1 mm apart). Resultant images are useful in the assessment of specific morphologic features such as alveolar bone height and width for implant site assessment, the inferior alveolar canal in relation to impacted mandibular molars, condylar surface and shape in the symptomatic TMJ or evaluation of pathological conditions affecting the jaws.

- *Multiplanar volume reformations:* Any multiplanar image can be "thickened" by increasing the number of adjacent voxels included in the slice. This creates an image that represents a specific volume of the patient. The simplest technique is adding the absorption values of adjacent voxels, to produce a "ray sum" image. This mode can be used to generate simulated panoramic images by increasing the slice thickness of curved planar reformatted images along the dental arch to 25–30 mm, comparable to the in focus image layer of panoramic radiographs. (Fig. 7.4B) Alternatively, plain projection images such as lateral cephalometric images can be created from full thickness (130–150 mm) perpendicular MPR images. In this case, such images can be exported and analyzed using third-party proprietary cephalometric software. Unlike conventional radiographs, these ray sum images are without magnification and are undistorted. Another thickening technique is maximum intensity projection (MIP). MIP images are achieved by displaying only the highest voxel value within a particular thickness. This mode produces a "pseudo" 3-D structure and is particularly useful in representing the surface morphology of the maxillofacial region. More complicated shaded surface displays and volume rendering algorithms can be applied to the entire thickness of the volumetric data set to provide 3-D reconstruction and presentation of data that can be interactively enhanced.

CBCT imaging provides clinicians with sub-millimetre spatial resolution images of high diagnostic quality with relatively short scanning times (10–70 seconds) and a reported radiation dose equivalent to that needed for 4 to 15 panoramic radiographs.

Terakado et al published the first cone-beam CT image of a TMJ, showing a single case of condylar fracture. In his study, he used Ortho-CT in evaluating the oral and maxillofacial region. The development of ortho cubic super-high resolution CT (Ortho-CT) optimized for dental diseases was started in 1992 in the Department of Radiology at Nihon University School of Dentistry. Development was completed in 1997, and its clinical application has already been reported. The radiation doses are about 1/30 of those of conventional X-ray CT and are about the same as those of rotational panoramic radiography. Sectional images can be obtained in any direction, at any tomographic layer, and at any interval within the range of the cylinder. Sections parallel to the dental arch (parallel sections), perpendicular to the dental arch (cross-sections), and horizontal sections are produced with a slice width of 1 mm at an interval of 1 mm. The representative images can be registered in a database and printed out.

In comparison with the conventional methods, the resolution was high in examining a small area, and the extent of the lesion and positional relationships with the maxillary sinus, mandibular canal, and proximal teeth could be examined. Because Ortho-CT can take high-resolution 3-dimensional images at any tomographic layer with only 1 exposure, it is useful for the diagnosis of diseases in the oral and maxillofacial region.

Honda et al presented the first study that systematically compared cone-beam CT and spiral CT of the TMJ, also estimating the diagnostic reliability based on a comparison of imaging findings with macroscopic observations. They found that both cone-beam CT and spiral CT were highly reliable for evaluation of the bony mandibular condyle. Being much cheaper and with considerably lower radiation dose in patient examinations, cone-beam CT is both a cost-effective and a dose-effective alternative diagnostic method for examination of the bony components of the TMJ.

A reconstruction technique was introduced in a report by Tsiklakis, which resulted in obtaining lateral and coronal CBCT images as well as 3-D reconstructions of the TMJ (Fig. 7.5). The technique is described as under:

The technique was used with a CBCT scanner operating with a maximum output of 110 kV and 10 mA, with 0.7 mm Al-equivalent filtration and a standard 14° cone-beam angle. The patient is placed in a supine position with the head within the circular gantry housing the X-ray tube and the detectors. Accurate positioning of the head is facilitated by the use of two light-beam markers. The vertical positioning light must be aligned with the mid-sagittal line of the patient, which helps keep the head of the patient centred with respect to the

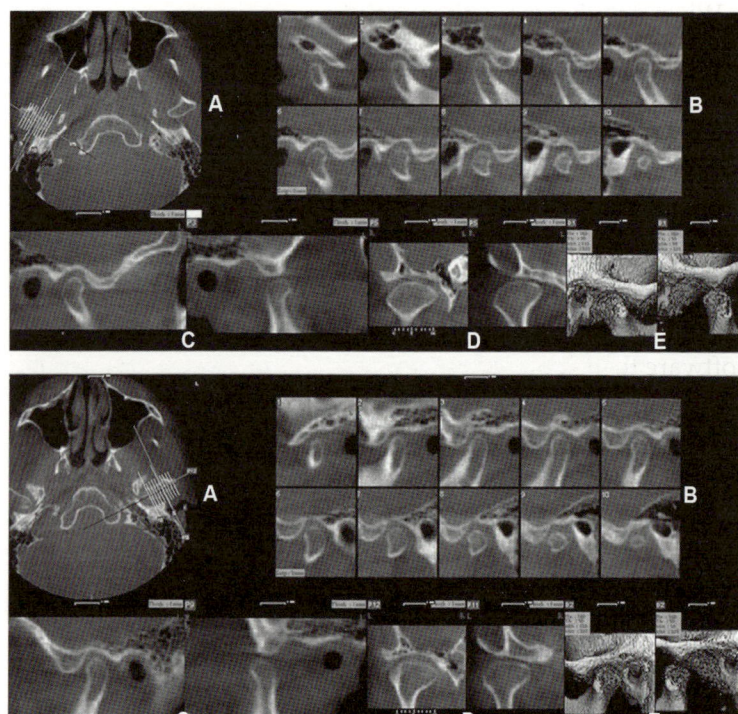

Figs 7.5 A to E: Film layout of a typical examination of the right and left temporomandibular joint. (A) Axial image, (B) lateral images perpendicular to the long axis of the condyle (closed mouth), (C) central lateral images (closed and open mouth), (D) coronal views parallel to the long axis of the condyle (closed and open mouth) and (E) three-dimensional reconstructions (closed and open mouth)

rotational axis. The lateral positioning light is centred at the level of the condyles, indicating the optimized centre of the reconstruction area. The X-ray tube-detectors system performs a 360° rotation around the head of the patient. Scanning time is 76s and the output is automatically adjusted during the 360° rotation according to tissue density, the so called "smart beam technology." If the range and type of movement of the condyle needs to be assessed, a second scanning of the patient takes place. The scanning procedure is the same only with the patient's mouth open. A bite block can be used to keep the mouth wide open.

When acquisition of the second raw data is completed, the patient may leave the examination room and the clinician is able to perform the primary reconstruction. The area of interest, in this case the TMJ, is defined and the software automatically generates a series of axial slices of 1 mm thickness (Fig. 7.6A).

One of the axial views is used as a reference view for secondary reconstruction. To orient the reconstruction according to the individual angle of the condyle, a line is traced that corresponds to the long axis of the examined condyle. This line also defines the most distal and medial point on the condyle that the secondary reconstruction will cover (Fig. 7.6B). The software then generates lateral slices perpendicular to the long axis of the condyle. The lateral views are reformatted images perpendicular to the plane of the axial views. Depending on the size of the condyle, eight to ten lateral views can be obtained, spaced 2 mm apart, thus covering the defined region of interest from the lateral to the medial pole (Fig. 7.5B).

In addition, since the centre of the condyle is defined during the previous steps, the lateral slice that corresponds to this central point is used as a reference lateral view, revealing the true position of the condyle in the fossa (Fig. 7.5C). The third step of the technique involves reconstruction of images parallel to the long axis of the condyle, leading to the acquisition of coronal slices of 2 mm thickness (Figs 7.5D and 7.7).

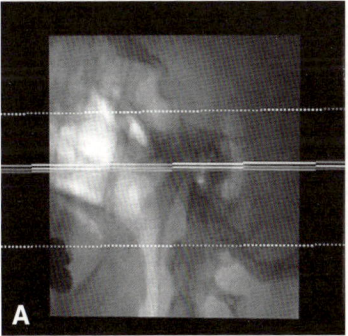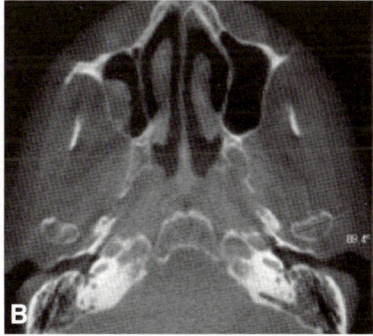

Figs 7.6A and B: (A) The area of interest (e.g. temporomandibular joint) is defined on the raw data. (B) axial image resulting from the primary reconstruction. The user traces a line that corresponds to the long axis of the examined condyle, defining simultaneously the most distal and medial point that the secondary reconstruction will cover

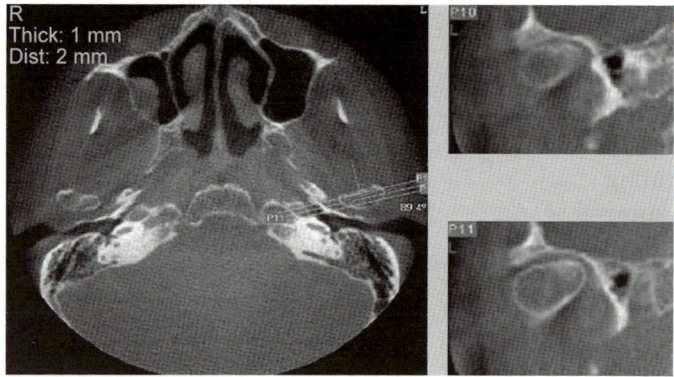

Fig. 7.7: Reconstruction of axial slices parallel to the long axis of the condyle; production of coronal slices of 2 mm thickness. The software also provides the option for 3-D reconstruction

In the open-mouth position the same procedure described above is performed. Central lateral and coronal views are generated as well as 3-D reconstruction images of the condyle, which is normally positioned in this case slightly over the tubercle, often resulting in better visualization of its body.

The technique described in this paper provides images that are obtained in planes parallel or perpendicular to the long axis of the condyle instead of the true anatomic coronal and sagittal planes. This results in high quality images of the bony components on all planes. Developmental and pathological changes can be detected using the lateral views. Furthermore, the central lateral view defines the true position of the condyle in the fossa, which often reveals possible dislocation of the disc in the joint.

Additional information on the condition of the surface of the condyle head can be obtained by the coronal views. Pathological changes that are potentially concealed in the lateral images may be revealed in the coronal views owing to their orientation being perpendicular to the lateral ones. The coronal views of the condyle obtained with conventional techniques, e.g. linear tomography or reverse Towne's, are of low image quality. Therefore, they are hardly included in the routine TMJ radiographic examination since they increased radiation risk for the patient without achieving significant diagnostic benefit.

On the other hand, the CBCT coronal views are of high image quality and are obtained within a few seconds without any additional irradiation of the patient. Finally, a 3-D reconstruction gives a general overview of the TMJ, sometimes valuable in cases with severe morphological abnormalities or for surgical planning.

Examining the joint with open mouth can be helpful in diagnosing internal derangement in the joint. The central lateral view gives information regarding the extent of translation of the condyle in the fossa. Furthermore, the coronal view in the open-mouth situation often leads to a clearer view of the condyle, since it translates slightly over the tubercle giving an unobstructed view of the condyle head. It should always be taken into consideration, however, that a second scanning with open mouth doubles the radiation dose for the patient; it should thus be performed only in cases where the additional diagnostic information outweighs the increased risk.

According to the manufacturer, owing to the use of the cone-shaped X-ray beam and the "smart beam technology", the absorbed dose from a CBCT scan is approximately equivalent to two to five panoramic exposures; however, this claim needs further investigation. Additionally, the CBCT scanning time of 76s is shorter than the time required for a conventional CT examination. This time is also shorter compared with conventional tomography. For instance, an exposure time of 56s is required to take just four lateral tomograms of a single TMJ using conventional spiral tomography.

In 2004 Honda et al studied usefulness of the limited cone-beam X-ray CT (3DX) (Morita Co., Japan) in measuring the thickness of the roof of the glenoid fossa (RGF) of the temporomandibular joint (TMJ). A commercially available 3DX system was used to image the TMJ of the cadaver specimens. A single 3608 scan collected projection data from a cylinder (height 30 mm; diameter 40 mm) for the image reconstruction. The exposure factors were 80 kVp, 2 mA and 17s. [7–10] Image data were quantified on a two-dimensional screen measuring 240 pixels in the vertical direction by 320 pixels in the horizontal direction, with each pixel quantified at 8 bits, and stored electronically. The image reconstruction took approximately 3 min and the distance between the images was 1 mm. The imaging dimensions were 30 mm in height (240 voxels) and 40 mm in diameter (320 voxels), with a voxel comprising square sides, each of which was 0.125 mm long. Owing to the cubic shape of the voxel, the resolution of the images was high and comparable in all directions. Figure 7.8 shows a block diagram of TMJ images from the 3DX in three planes: oblique sagittal, oblique coronal and axial, all obtained during one exposure. The thinnest area of the glenoid fossa was identified among the multiple slices on the monitor and a 3DX-image program was used to measure the thickness.

Figure 7.9 shows the thinnest RGF examined. In this specimen, the mandibular condyle was normal, the average 3DX-image tool measurement was 0.69 mm and the average micrometer measurement was 0.84 mm. Figure 7.10 shows the thickest RGF examined. In this specimen, the mandibular condyle showed an osteophyte formation, the average 3DX-image tool measurement was 1.70 mm and the average micrometer measurement was 1.86 mm. The average macroscopic examination measurement was 1.37 mm (range:

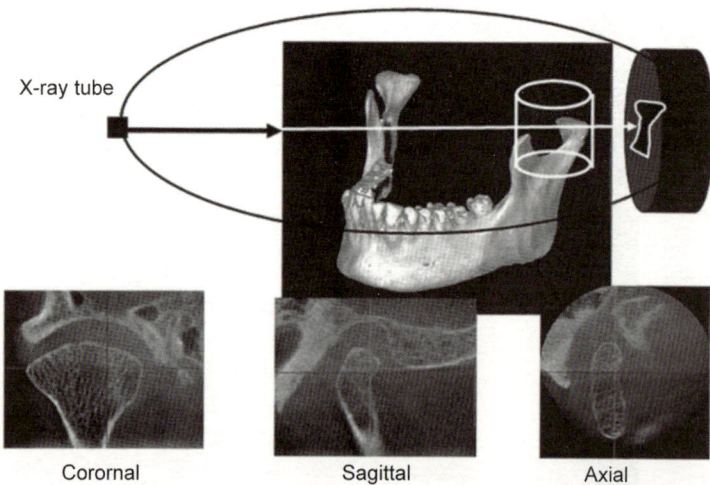

X-ray tube

Corornal   Sagittal   Axial

Fig. 7.8: Block diagram of the cone-beam CT (3DX). Temporomandibular joint images from the 3DX in three planes: oblique sagittal, oblique coronal and axial; obtained during one exposure. The imaging dimensions were 30 mm in height (240 voxels) and 40 mm in diameter (320 voxels), with a voxel comprising square sides, each of which was 0.125 mm long

0.55–3.6 mm) and the average 3DX image measurement was 1.22 mm (range: 0.51–3.0 mm). Skin dose comparisons between conventional CT and the 3DX system used in this study showed that a much lower dose is needed for 3DX (1.19 mSv) than for helical-CT (160 mSv). This suggests that the 3DX system is more useful for diagnostic analysis of hard tissue in dentistry and otology than conventional CT techniques. It was concluded that the 3DX is useful for clinical applications in TMJ diagnosis based on its accuracy of measurements and decreased radiation compared with helical CT.

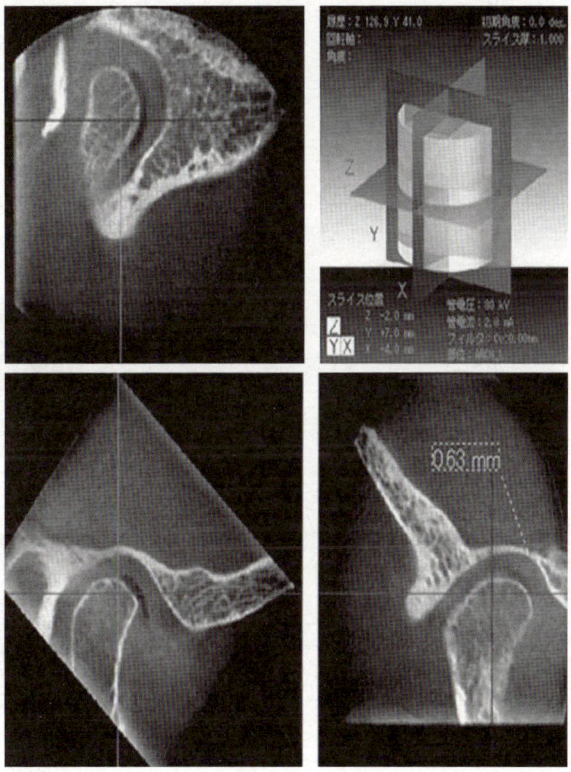

Fig. 7.9: The thinnest measurement of the roof of the glenoid fossa. The mandibular condyle was normal, the first cone-beam CT (3DX)-image tool measurement was 0.63 mm and the first digimatic outside micrometer measurement was 0.65 mm

In 2006 Honda et al conducted another study to evaluate the usefulness of the limited cone-beam CT and helical computed tomography (helical CT) for the detection of osseous abnormalities of the mandibular condyle, using macroscopic observations. Twenty-one temporomandibular joint autopsy specimens underwent imaging with 3DX and helical CT. The specimens were macroscopically evaluated for cortical erosion or osteophytosis and sclerosis. The images were independently assessed for the same osseous abnormalities. Observations with the two imaging modalities were compared with the

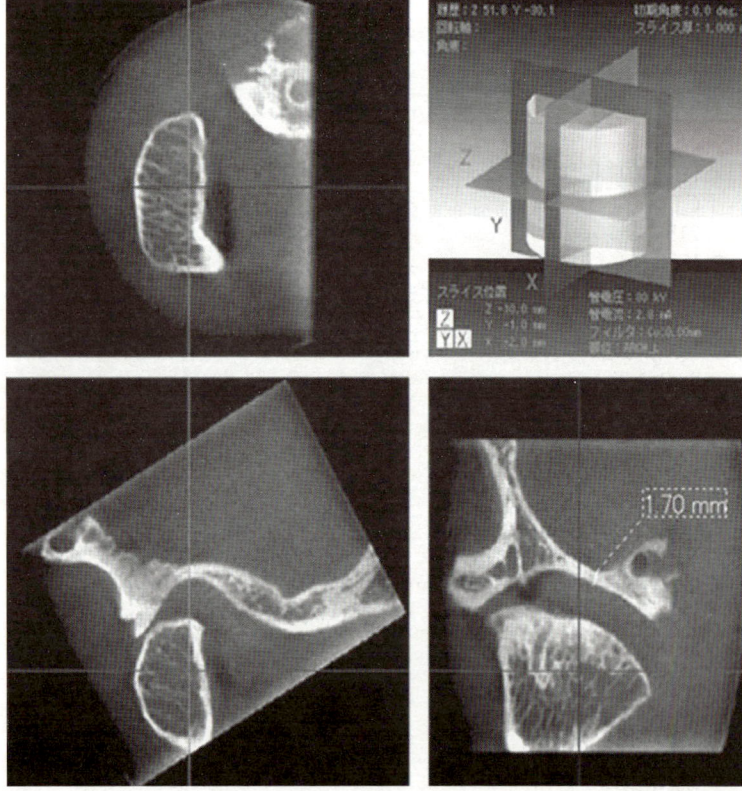

Fig. 7.10: The thickest measurement of roof of the glenoid fossa. The mandibular condyle showed an osteophyte formation, the first cone-beam CT (3DX)-image tool measurement was 1.70 mm and the first micrometer measurement was 1.75 mm

macroscopic observations using the McNemar test. Results showed macroscopic observations, 10 of the 21 mandibular condyles and one fossa showed osseous abnormalities. 3DX detected abnormalities in eight of these condyles and helical CT identified abnormalities in seven, giving a sensitivity of 0.80 for 3DX and 0.70 for helical CT. The specificity of the condyle assessment was 1.0 for both 3DX and helical CT and hence, the accuracy was 0.90 and 0.86, respectively. No significant differences were detected between the 3DX and helical CT for assessment of osseous abnormalities of the mandibular condyle (P ¼ 0.286). They concluded that the cone-beam CT equipment 3DX is a dose-effective and a cost-effective alternative to helical CT for the diagnostic evaluation of osseous abnormalities of the mandibular condyle.

BIBLIOGRAPHY

1. Hu H, He HD, Foley WD, Fox SH. Four multidetector-row helical CT: image quality and volume coverage speed. *Radiology* 2000; 215(1):55–62.
2. K Honda, Y Arai, M Kashima, Y Takana, K Sawada, K Ejima, K Iwai. Evaluation of the usefulness of the limited cone-beam CT (3DX) in the assessment of the thickness of the roof of the glenoid fossa of the temporomandibular joint. Dentomaxillofacial Radiology 2004; 33:391–5.
3. K Honda, TA Larheim, K Maruhashi, K Matsumoto, K Iwai. Osseous abnormalities of the mandibular condyle: diagnostic reliability of cone-beam computed tomography compared with helical computed tomography based on an autopsy material. Dentomaxillofacial Radiology 2006; 35:152–7.
4. Kishi K, Hasegawa I, Shigehara H, et al.Clinical application of 3-D C T and 3-D plastic model in the maxillo-facial region. Oral Radiol 1997;13: 83–92.
5. K Tsiklakis, K Syriopoulos, HC Stamatakis. Radiographic examination of the temporomandibular joint using cone-beam computed tomography. Dentomaxillofacial Radiology 2004; 33:196–201.
6. Terakado M, Hashimoto K, Arai Y, Honda M, Sekiwa T, Sato H. Diagnostic imaging with newly developed ortho cubic super-high resolution computed tomography (Ortho-CT). Oral Surg Oral Med Oral Pathol Oral Radiol Endo 2000; 89:509–18.
7. William C. Scarfe, Allan G. Farman, Predag Sukovic: Clinical Applications of Cone-Beam Computed Tomography in Dental Practice J Can Dent Assoc 2006; 72 (1):75–80.

Magnetic Resonance Imaging

Magnetic resonance imaging (MRI) is a noninvasive technique that uses a magnetic field and radiofrequency pulses instead of ionizing radiation to produce the images. In general, MRI is a more expensive examination because of the cost of the equipment, facilities, staffing and replacement cryogens for the magnet. MR imaging has been used to image the TMJ since 1984, and imaging quality has continuously improved since that time. Information available about the TMJ from MRI includes the location of the disk in both open and closed mouth positions at multiple levels through the joint. Mediolateral and rotational displacements can be detected, as well as the straight anterior displacements. However, disk perforations and capsular tears are better detected with arthrography. Although the detail of the osseous structures is not as well depicted as with conventional tomography or CT, information on bony contours and cortical outline is available with MRI. In addition, abnormalities within the bone marrow of the condyle and within the muscles and surrounding soft tissues can be detected. Other information obtainable includes the presence of soft tissue in growths, fibrosis and joint effusion, the latter of which has been correlated to pain in the joint. A recent report has demonstrated that the accuracy of MRI with respect to disk position may reach 95%. However, the diagnostic quality of these examinations can vary widely between institutions, depending on the experience level of both the technologists and the radiologists who interpret the examination, as well as the field strength of the magnet, surface coils and software of the MR imager itself.

HISTORY OF MRI IN BRIEF

1. Felix Bloch and Edward Purcell, discovered the magnetic resonance phenomenon independently in 1946.
2. In the period between 1950 and 1970, NMR was developed and used for chemical and physical molecular analysis.
3. In 1971 *Raymond Damadian* showed that the nuclear magnetic relaxation times of tissues and tumors differed, thus motivating scientists to consider magnetic resonance for the detection of disease.
4. In 1973 Magnetic resonance imaging was first demonstrated on small test tube samples by *Paul Lauterbur.*
5. In 1975 *Richard Ernst* proposed magnetic resonance imaging using phase and frequency encoding, and the Fourier Transform. This technique is the basis of current MRI techniques.
6. In 1977, *Raymond Damadian* demonstrated MRI of the whole body. In the same year, *Peter Mansfield* developed the echo-planar imaging (EPI) technique.
7. *Edelstein and coworkers* demonstrated imaging of the body using Ernst's technique in 1980.
8. By 1986, the imaging time was reduced to about five seconds, without sacrificing too much image quality.
9. In 1987 echo-planar imaging was used to perform real-time movie imaging of a single cardiac cycle.
10. In 1991, *Richard Ernst* was rewarded for his achievements in pulsed Fourier Transform NMR and MRI.
11. In 1993 functional MRI (fMRI) was developed.
12. In 1994, researchers at the State University of New York at Stony Brook and Princeton University demonstrated the imaging of hyperpolarized 129Xe gas for respiration studies. MRI is clearly a young, but growing science.
13. In 1999, MagneVu developed the first truly portable MRI technology and made MRI technology available in the office of the clinician.

IMAGING PRINCIPLES

In contrast to other imaging techniques, magnetic resonance imaging uses nonionizing radiation from the radiofrequency (RF) band of the electromagnetic spectrum. To produce an MR image, the patient is placed inside a large magnet, which induces a relatively strong external magnetic field. This causes the nuclei of many atoms in the body, including hydrogen, to align themselves with the magnetic field. After application of an RF signal, energy is released from the body, detected, and used to construct the MR image by computer. The high contrast sensitivity of MRI to tissue differences and the absence of radiation exposure are the main advantages of MRI over CT.

The theory of MRI is based on the magnetic properties of an atom. Atomic nuclei spin about their axes much as the earth spins about its axis. In addition, individual protons and neutrons are evenly paired; the spin of each nucleon cancels that of another, producing a net spin of zero. In nuclei that contain an unpaired proton or neutron, a net spin is created. Because spin is associated with an electrical charge, a magnetic field is generated in nuclei with unpaired nucleons, causing these nuclei to act as magnets with north and south poles (magnetic dipoles).

The nucleus of the element hydrogen contains a single, unpaired proton, and therefore acts as a magnetic dipole. A sample containing many hydrogen atoms would find these magnetic dipoles to be oriented randomly. This results in a total magnetization for the sample of zero (Fig. 8.1).

In this natural state, if an external magnetic field is applied to the sample, all the hydrogen nuclear axes line up in the direction of the magnetic field, producing a quantity of net magnetization.

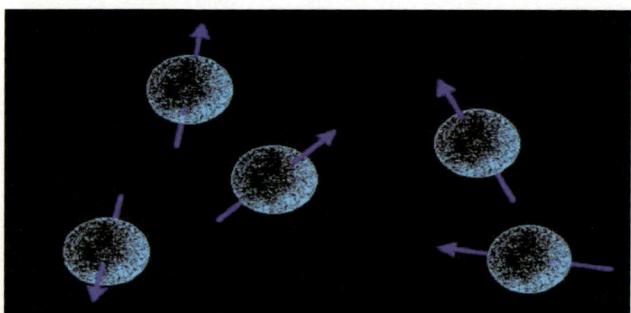

Fig. 8.1: A sample of hydrogen nuclei with net spins showing these dipoles to be randomly oriented

However, not all north poles point in the same direction. Rather, two states are possible: *spin up*, which parallels the external magnetic field, and *spin down*, which is antiparallel with the field (Fig. 8.2). The combined effect of these two energy states is a weak net magnetic moment, or *magnetization vector (Mv)*. More energy is required to align antiparallel with the magnetic field, therefore, these hydrogen nuclei are considered to be at a higher energy state than those parallel with the field. Nuclei can be made to undergo transition from one energy state to another by absorbing or releasing a certain quantity of energy. Energy required for transition from the lower to the higher, or from higher to the lower energy level can be supplied or recovered in the form of electromagnetic energy in the RF portion of the electromagnetic spectrum. The transition from one energy level to another is called *resonance*.

When an external magnetic field is applied to a sample of nuclei, their north and south poles do not align exactly with the direction of the magnetic field. The axes of spinning protons actually oscillate or wobble with a slight tilt from a position absolutely parallel with the flux of external magnet. This tilting or wobbling, called *precession*, is similar to that of a spinning toy top, which does not spin in a perfectly upright position as it slows down, because of the effect of the earth's gravitational field. The axis of the spinning top wobbles about the direction of the local gravitational field, and the axis of spinning proton wobbles (or precesses) about the magnetic field. Because of the spin up and spin down states, the spinning protons precess

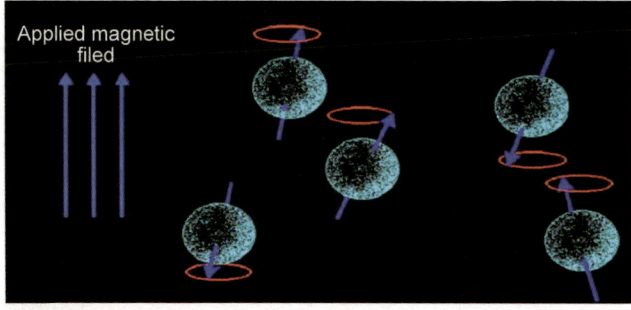

Fig. 8.2: Spin up and spin down state of hydrogen atoms in case of applied magnetic field

together in the direction of their spin states, which can be visualized as two cones placed end to end.

The rate or frequency of the precession is called the ***resonant or Larmour frequency***. It depends on the species of nucleus and is proportional to the strength of the external magnetic field. The Larmor frequency of hydrogen is 42.58 MHz in a magnetic field of 1 Tesla (T). One tesla is 10,000 times the earth's magnetic field. The magnetic field strengths used for MR imaging range from 0.1 to 4.0 T.

When energy in the form of an electromagnetic wave in the radiofrequency range from an RF antenna coil is directed to tissue with protons (hydrogen nuclei) that are aligned in the Z-axis by an external static magnetic field (by the imaging magnet), the protons in the tissue that have a Larmor frequency matching that of an electromagnetic wave absorb energy and shift or rotate away from the direction induced by the imaging magnet. The longer the RF impulse is applied, the greater the angle of rotation. If the pulse is of sufficient intensity (duration), it will rotate the net tissue magnetization vector into the transverse plane (XY plane), which is perpendicular to longitudinal alignment (Z axis), and cause all the protons to precess in phase. This is referred to as a ***90-degree RF pulse or a flip angle 90-degrees***. During an MR imaging sequence, many RF pulses with different intensities can be used, along with different times between repetitions of the pulse. The net magnetization of the tissue in the transverse plane and the amount of transverse magnetization that exists at the termination of the RF pulse are equal to the amount of longitudinal magnetization that existed just before the pulse. Both are directly proportional to the strength of the static magnetic field and the number of hydrogen nuclei (protons) present in the tissue. At this precise moment, a maximal RF signal is induced in a receiver coil. The magnitude of this signal represents information about the overall concentration of hydrogen nuclei (proton density) in a sample of tissue or about the number of hydrogen nuclei in a sample of different types of tissue. This signal depends not only on the presence or absence of hydrogen but also on the degree to which hydrogen is bound within a molecule. Tightly bound hydrogen atoms, such as those present in bone, do not align themselves with the external magnetic field and do not produce a usable signal. Loosely bound or mobile hydrogen atoms such as those present in soft tissues and liquids tilt and align to produce a detectable signal. The measure of the concentration of loosely bound hydrogen nuclei available to create the signal is referred to as *proton density or spin density* of the tissue in question. The higher the concentration of these nuclei of loosely bound hydrogen atoms the stronger the net magnetization at equilibrium and at all degrees of excitement, the more intense the recovered signal, and the lighter the MR image.

As soon as the radiowaves (the resonant RF pulse) are turned off, two events occur simultaneously; the radiation of energy and the return of the nuclei to their original spin state at a lower energy. This process is called *relaxation*, and the energy loss is detected as a signal, which is called *free induction decay (FID).*

First, the nuclei in transverse alignment begin to realign themselves with the main magnetic field (i.e. to relax), and net magnetization regrows to the original longitudinal orientation. Relaxation is accomplished by a transfer of energy from individual hydrogen nuclei (spin) to the surrounding molecules (lattice). The time constant that describes the rate at which net magnetization returns to equilibrium by transfer of energy is called the T1 relaxation time or spin lattice relaxation time. T1 varies with different tissues and the ability of nuclei to transfer their excess energy to their environment. A T1 weighted image is produced by a short repetition time between RF pulses and a short signal recovery time. Because T1 is an exponential growth time constant, a tissue with a short T1 produces an intense MR signal, displayed as bright white in a T1 weighted image. A tissue with a long T1 produces a low intensity signal and appears dark in the MR image.

Second, the magnetic moments of adjacent hydrogen nuclei begin to interfere with one another; this causes the nuclei to diphase, with a resultant loss of transverse magnetization. The time constant that describes the rate of loss of transverse magnetization is called T2 relaxation time or transverse (spin-spin) relaxation time. The transverse magnetization rapidly decays to zero, as do the amplitude and duration of the detected radiosignal. A T2 weighted image is acquired using a long repetition time between RF pulses and a long signal recovery time. A tissue with a long T2 produces a high intensity signal and is bright in the image. One with a short T2 produces a low intensity signal and is dark in the image. The FID relates signal intensity to time. A mathematical technique called the *Fourier transform* converts the relationship of signal intensity versus time to signal intensity versus resonant frequency, transforming the oscillating FID signal to a pulse of energy (current), the MR signal. When FIDs are received from a mixture of tissues, as in a case when a section of the body is examined, each volume of tissue generates a different radio signal at different frequencies. The antenna does not separate the individual signals; rather, they are assumed to form a complex FID signal. The Fourier transform also separated the complex FID signal from the different tissues into its various frequency components. This procedure is coupled with reconstruction techniques similar to those in CT to produce diagnostic images.

Image contrast among the various tissues in the body is manipulated in MRI by varying the rate at which the RF pulses are transmitted.

T1 Weighted Images

- A short repetition time (TR) of 500 msec between pulses and a short echo or signal recovery time (TE) of 20 msec produces a T1 weighted image.

- T1 weighted images are fat images because fat has the shortest T1 relaxation time and the highest signal relative to the other tissues and thus appears bright in the image.

- High anatomic detail is possible in this type of image because of good image contrast.

- T1 weighted images are useful for depicting small anatomic regions (e.g. TMJ) where high spatial resolution is required.

A long repetition time of 2000 msec and a long echo or signal recovery time of 80 msec produces a T2 weighted image.

- T2 weighted images are called *water images* because water has the longest T2 relaxation time and thus appear bright in the image.

- T2 weighting are most commonly used when the practitioner is looking for inflammatory or other pathologic changes.

Localization of the MR image to a specific part of the body (selecting a slice) and the ability to create a three-dimensional image depend on the fact that the Larmor frequency of a nucleus is governed in part by the strength of the external magnetic field. When this strength is changed in a gradient across a body of tissue (selectively exciting the image slice), the Larmor frequency of individual nuclei or groups of nuclei (voxels) in the gradient also changes. Three electromagnetic coils within the bore of the imaging magnet produce this magnetic gradient. The coils surround the patient and produce magnetic influx in three orthogonal or right angle directions to delineate individual volumes of tissues (voxels), which are subjected to magnetic fields of unique strength.

Partitioning the local magnetic fields tunes all the hydrogen protons in a particular voxel to the same resonant frequency. This is called *selective excitation*. When an RF pulse with a range of frequencies is applied, a voxel of tissue tuned to one frequency is excited; when the RF radiation is terminated, the excited voxel radiates that distinctive frequency, identifying and localizing it. The bandwidth or spectrum of frequencies of the RF pulse and the magnitude of the slice selecting gradient determine the slice thickness. Slice thickness can be reduced by increasing gradient strength or decreasing the RF bandwidth (frequency range).

MAGNETIC FIELD STRENGTH AND COMPARISON WITH CT

Scanners with magnetic field strengths ranging from 0.05 to 2 Tesla are currently in clinical use; however, studies that compare the image quality of these scanners with different magnetic field strengths are scarce. One study compared images from two different scanners obtained with equal acquisition time and demonstrated significantly better image quality with the high-field system. Although the lower image quality of the 0.3 Tesla scanner could be somewhat compensated for by increasing the acquisition time (the number of excitations) by a factor of about 4, in clinical work this increases the risk of motion artifact.

MRI OF TEMPOROMANDIBULAR JOINT

Normal MRI Anatomy

T1 weighted images are most valuable for depicting normal TMJ anatomy. These images show the cortical bone as dark to black, with the articular disc and dense fascia more black to grey. Normal muscles appear grey, with fat and bone marrow almost white. The osseous TMJ components include the mandibular condyle, the glenoid fossa and the articular eminence. They appear white with a black outline. The osseous boundaries include the anterior slope of the articular eminence, the tympanic portion of the temporal bone posteriorly, and the rest of the zygomatic arch laterally, and the temporal process medially.

The fibrocartilagenous disc lies interposed between the mandibular condyle and the temporal joint compartment. It measures approximately 20–25 mm and is thinner in the center than at the periphery, forming a biconcave configuration. On the MRI the edges are of low signal intensity (black) while the middle being of somewhat higher intensity (grey).

The bilaminar zone gives signal of intermediate intensity because of its fat and water content which produces a faint demarcation between the posterior disc and the bilaminar zone, although the demarcation may be absent or diminished in abnormally positioned discs.

The muscle most closely associated with TMJ is the lateral pterygoid muscle. The superior belly of lateral pterygoid muscle attaches to the anterior border of articular disc; the inferior belly attaches directly to the pterygoid fovea of mandibular condyle. Since muscles have intermediate signal intensity, they are distinguishable from the lower signal intensity of the articular disc. The fascial sheet containing fat that cover the lateral pterygoid muscles are noted to be white or light grey than the muscles. MRI studies have clearly identified the boundary between the disc and the retrodiscal area in subjects with symptomatic and asymptomatic TMJs. Katz-berg et al reported that the retrodiscal tissue has a bright signal in relation to the posterior band of disc on T1 or proton density images due to the rich network of fatty tissue or possibly, the higher water content due to the vascularity. Pseudodynamic MR study has shown that wider the mouth opening, the higher the intensity in the retrodiscal tissue. These findings reflect the blood pumping function of the retrodiscal tissue. One of the functional disorders of TMJ is internal derangement, i.e. derangement of the condyle disc complex.

The most common symptoms of internal derangements of TMJ are pain, muscular tenderness, a clicking or popping sensation within the joint, headache, earache and limited ability to open the jaw.

The severity of internal derangement can be graded according to the morphology of the disc:

Grade 1 (anterior disc displacement with reduction): An anteriorly displaced disc that maintains its normal biconcave configuration.

Grade 2 (anterior disc displacement without reduction): An anteriorly displaced disc which does not have normal morphology.

Draze and Enzamann gave criteria for the degree of disc anterior disc displacement as follows:

0–10–normal disc position (no disc displacement)

11–30–slight anterior disc displacement (early disc reduction)

31–50–mild anterior disc displacement (medium disc reduction)

51–80–moderate anterior disc displacement (late disc reduction)

Over 80–severe anterior disc displacement (without disc reduction)

Schmitter et al conducted a study on 100 TMJ. The objectives of the study were, on the one hand, to assess the extent to which the quality of sagittal MR images of the TMJ influences inter-rater agreement between different groups of raters and, on the other hand, to evaluate inter-rater agreement with respect to the assessment of image quality.

Initial pilot scans were obtained in the closed-mouth and opened-mouth positions to detect the condyles in the various functional positions. On the axial pilot images, the slices of the diagnostic sequences were angulated vertical to the mandibular condyle, so that the first slice consisted of the lateral portion of the condyle and the fifth slice consisted of the medial portion of the condyle (Fig. 8.3).

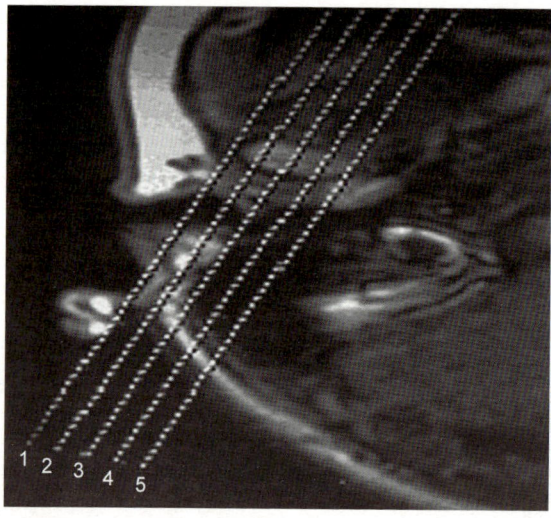

Fig. 8.3: An initial pilot scan used to detect the position of the condyles with the patient's mouth closed

Image quality was assessed subjectively. No assessment criteria were provided. The raters used a rating scale for image quality that ranged from 0 (poor) to 5 (very good). The images were then assigned to one of two categories according to the rating results. Category II (moderate to poor quality, Fig. 8.4)

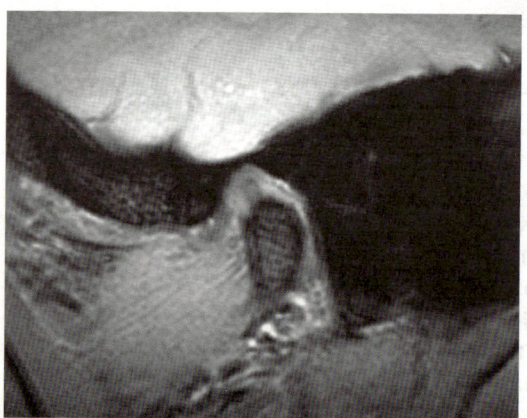

Fig. 8.4: Example of an MRI scan (category II; mean rating 2.25) on which the dentists and radiologists were not in agreement

consisted of images with a rating of 3 or less, while category I (good image quality, Fig. 8.5) was used for images with a rating of 4 or 5. They concluded that good image quality can enhance inter-rater agreement. If a poor quality image is analysed, image quality should be taken into consideration in the evaluation. In addition, subjective criteria that are carefully and critically applied may be used for quality assessment instead of objective criteria. Last but not least, in addition to quality assurance, calibration of raters seems to be useful to achieve better reliability for all criteria.

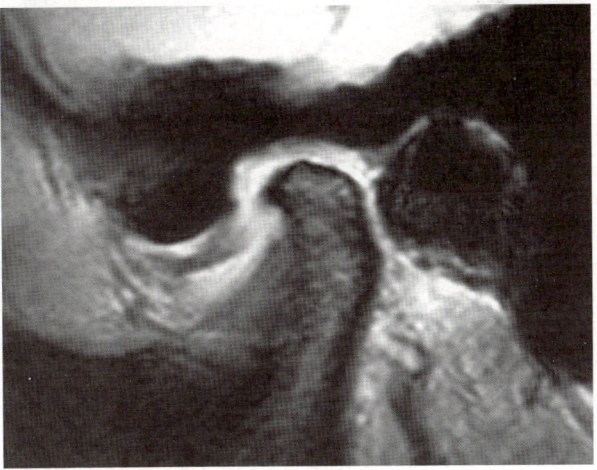

Fig. 8.5: Example of an MRI scan (category I; mean rating 4.5) on which all four raters were in complete agreement

Disk displacement and arthrosis are the most common findings on MR images of the temporomandibular joint (TMJ) in patients with signs and symptoms of a TMJ disorder. Disk displacement is defined as an abnormal relationship between the disk and mandibular condyle involving an anterior, medial, or lateral displacement of the disk from its normal position superior to the condyle. These abnormalities are often but not always associated with pain. Clinically, it's noted that MR evidence of joint effusion is frequently present in painful joints with disk displacement but rarely in normal joints. If a strong association between the presence of joint effusion and an abnormal and painful joint could be established, this could be the basis for valuable additional diagnostic information from MR imaging of the TMJ.

Westesson and Brook conducted a study to systematically correlate MR findings of joint effusion with different stages of disk displacement, arthrosis, and the clinical symptom of pain. They found MR evidence of joint effusion in about 30% of joints in a consecutive series of patients referred for MR imaging of the TMJ because of signs and symptoms of TMJ disorders. The association between MR evidence of joint effusion and joint pain was highly significant. The percentage of joints with joint effusion was greater in patients with the more advanced stages of disk displacement (displacement without reduction) than in those with the earlier stage (disk displacement with reduction). The prevalence of joint effusion was even lower in joints with arthrosis. These results indicate that joint effusion is associated with painful disk displacement.

The results of the study further emphasize that MR imaging is a valuable tool for imaging abnormalities of the TMJ in patients who have clinical signs and symptoms of disk displacement. The high prevalence of joint effusion and the strong association between effusion and joint pain make the diagnostic information obtained with the use of MR imaging valuable. Thus, if joint effusion is seen in an abnormal joint, it appears likely that this joint has some degree of pain. This information is valuable to both the clinician and the radiologist for confirming that the joint is abnormal. For these reasons, it seems wise to routinely include T2-weighted images in an MR study of the TMJ. On T2-weighted images, the arthrographic effect caused by joint effusion occasionally helped in defining the extent of a perforation of the posterior disk attachment. This is another reason to obtain T2-weighted images.

Dennis P Haley et al conducted a study to evaluate the relationship between TMJ pain and clinical *vs* MRI findings. The results of this study suggest that TMJ disc displacement was not significantly related to a patient's complaint of TMJ pain. MRI-depicted effusions were significantly related to the presence of TMJ pain. The authors recommend that clinicians should not use MRI-depicted effusions to assess for TMJ pain because of the large number of false-positive and false-negative findings, as well as the significant costs associated with conducting an MRI examination. This study indicates that TMJ palpation that elicits a complaint of pain that duplicates the patient's initial pain complaint is superior to MRI as an indicator that the TMJ is the source of the pain.

Sharon et al suggested that MRI has also been claimed to detect avascular necrosis of the condylar head and myxoid degeneration of the disk, although the significance of these findings is controversial. In patients with inflammatory arthritides, MRI has been shown to demonstrate disk destruction. With gadolinium used as a contrast agent, pannus formation can be detected in patients with active rheumatoid or other inflammatory arthritides. Because soft tissue alterations are likely to cause these symptoms, MRI is recommended to evaluate the condition of the disk. Initially panoramic or tomographic imaging is suggested to evaluate for osseous changes. MRI is indicated if there is concern about disk displacement or other soft tissue abnormalities.

Sano and Westesson analyze if there was an association between the degree of pain and the T2 signal intensity from the retrodiscal tissue on MR images. Results of this study indicate a slightly increased T2 weighted MR signal from the retrodiscal tissue in painful joints when compared with non-painful joints. The signal intensity tended to be higher in the more painful joints. This may indicate a higher degree of vascularity in the retrodiscal tissue in the painful joints compared with the nonpainful joints.

They conclude that the T2 signal intensity from the retrodiscal tissue is higher in painful than in nonpainful joints. This might be related to increased vascularity in this tissue in painful joints.

In an article based on a sample of 123 TMJs, however, Adame and colleagues failed to relate TMJ pain to TMJ effusion. They described TMJ effusion as being related to the MRI finding of ID and OA.

Further, Murakami and colleagues studied high signal intensity and various pain levels in patients with unilateral TMJ painful closed locking. Data showed that there was no significant statistical correlation between pain levels and the presence of high signals. This study disclosed that the MRI detection of high signal intensity in the closed locking TMJ did not directly relate to the presence of TMJ pain nor the increased pain level.

Tsukasa Sano et al, analyze the relationship between abnormal bone marrow of the mandibular condyle and osteoarthritis. Study was based on MR images of 74 joints in 74 patients referred for MR imaging of the temporomandibular joint (TMJ) because of TMJ pain and dysfunction. Thirty-seven joints in 37 patients were selected because each showed MR evidence of a bone marrow abnormality such as marrow edema, marrow sclerosis, or a combination of edema and sclerosis. Osteoarthritis was seen in 22 of the 37 joints with bone marrow abnormalities, whereas the remaining 15 joints with bone marrow abnormalities had no MR evidence of osteoarthritis.

The combination of findings suggestive of edema and sclerosis was more frequently seen in joints demonstrating evidence of osteoarthritis than in joints without osteoarthritis Edema of the bone marrow without sclerosis, on the other hand, was more frequently seen in the joints without osteoarthritis.

They conclude that abnormal bone marrow of the mandibular condyle can occur separately from osteoarthritis; nearly one half of the joints with magnetic resonance evidence of abnormal bone marrow did not have any evident osteoarthritis.

Abnormal bone marrow may therefore initially represent a separate disease entity. Over time, secondary osteoarthritis probably develops in joints with initial bone marrow abnormalities. A clinical correlation of MRI findings of internal derangements of temporomandibular joint was given by Yilmaz and Toller in 2002 and reported that MRI should be used for surgical planning and in difficult cases to diagnose pathological conditions of the TMJ.

Sener and Akgunlu studied the differences between magnetic resonance imaging characteristics of anterior disc displacement with reduction (ADDWR) and without reduction. In his study the proportion of the sideways displacement was greater in ADDWR. Furthermore, the proportion of medial displacement was also greater in ADDWR. Medial displacement occurring more frequently than lateral displacement may be associated with the force of muscles that are attached to disc. It has been speculated that one reason for medial disc displacement is muscle spasm of the superior belly of the lateral pterygoid muscle.

On MRI, degenerative changes, effusion, the position, morphology and signal intensity of disc, scar tissue, osteonecrosis and condylar mobility were evaluated. They stated that as the dysfunction progresses, the disc become more deformed and may alter signal intensity, develop scar tissues and osteonecrosis. The diagnosis of ADDR and ADDWR was made on the MR images according to Larheim. In ADDR, the posterior band of the disc was anterior to the superior portion of the condylar head in the closed mouth position but the disc was located between the articular eminence and superior portion of the condylar head in the open mouth position. In ADDWR, the posterior band of the disc was anterior to the superior part of the condylar head both on closed and open mouth positions. Sideways displacements (in addition to anterior displacement) were classified into lateral and medial displacements, determined by a bulging of the articular disc laterally or medially on coronal images according to Katzberg and Westesson (Figs 8.6 and 8.7).

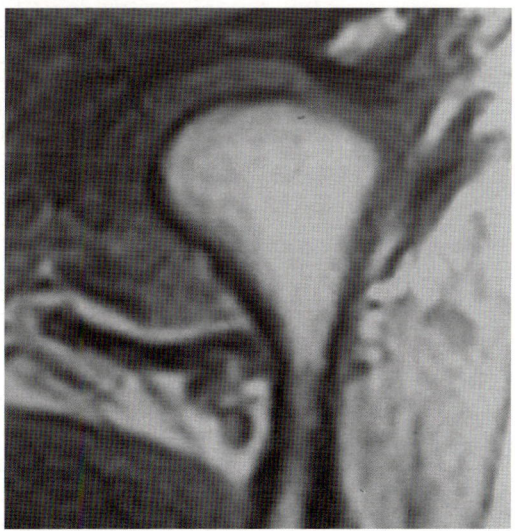

Fig. 8.6: MRI showing medial displacement in a case with anterior disc displacement with reduction (ADDR)

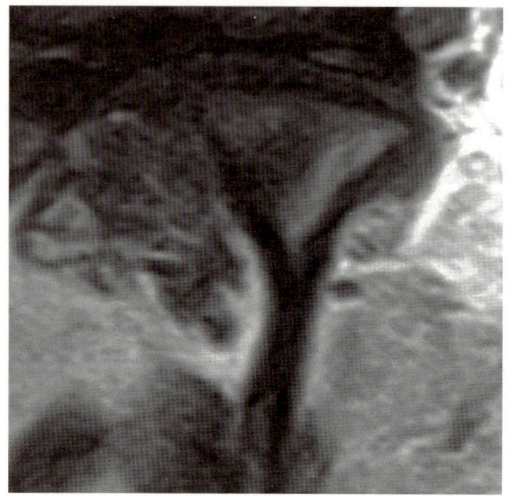

Fig. 8.7: MRI showing lateral displacement in a case with anterior disc displacement without reduction (ADDWR)

Erosion, flattening and osteophytes of the articular surfaces on coronal images are referred to as degenerative changes according to Katzberg and Westesson, (Figs 8.8 and 8.9) Larheim. The hyperintense areas on T2 weighted images are

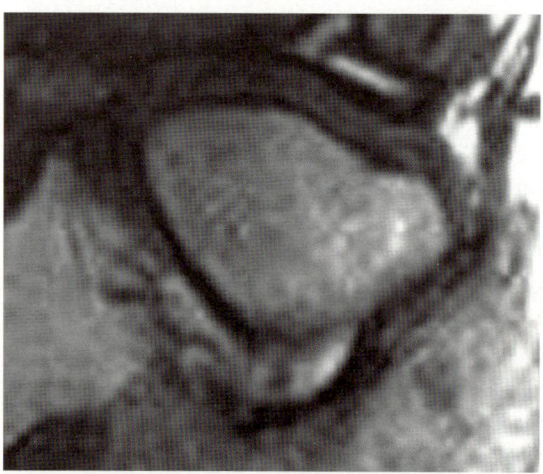

Fig. 8.8: MRI showing degenerative changes in a case with anterior disc displacement without reduction (ADDWR)

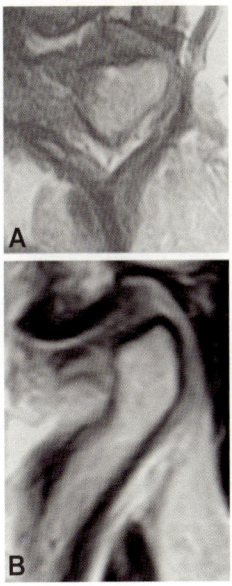

Figs 8.9A and B: (A) Coronal and (B) sagittal MR images showing degenerative change in a case with anterior disc displacement with reduction (ADDR)

described as effusion according to Rudisch et al and Adame et al (Figs 8.10 and 8.11).

Biconcave, bow-tie configurations of the disc were accepted as normal disc morphology according to Dijkgraaf et al, Katzberg and Westesson and Helms et al Morphological changes were classified into: elongation (thinning) (Fig. 8.12), thickening of posterior band (Fig. 8.13) and flexion (folding) (Fig. 8.14). The intermediate–low signal intensities were accepted as normal for the articular disc according to Helms et al. The changes in the signal intensity were classified into increased signal intensity (Fig. 8.12) or decreased signal intensity (Fig. 8.14).

On maximal opening of the mouth, hypermobility was diagnosed if the head of the condyle was in front of the articular eminence, according to Gynther et al and Shorey and Campbell (Figs 8.11 and 8.15)

Emshoff, Brandlmaier and colleagues conducted a study to evaluate whether TMJ pain disorder subgroups may be related

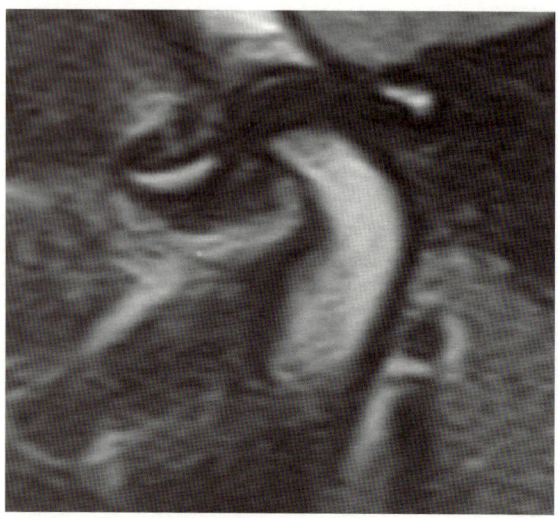

Fig. 8.10: MRI showing advanced effusion in a case with anterior disc displacement without reduction (ADDWR)

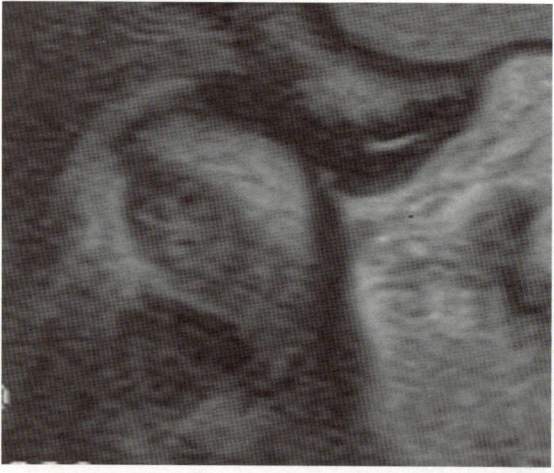

Fig. 8.11: MRI showing subluxation and minimal effusion in a case with anterior disc displacement with reduction (ADDR)

to MRI diagnoses of TMJ ID, OA, effusion and bone marrow edema, as well as to analyze whether common MRI features such as disk displacement; Osteoarthritis; effusion; and bone

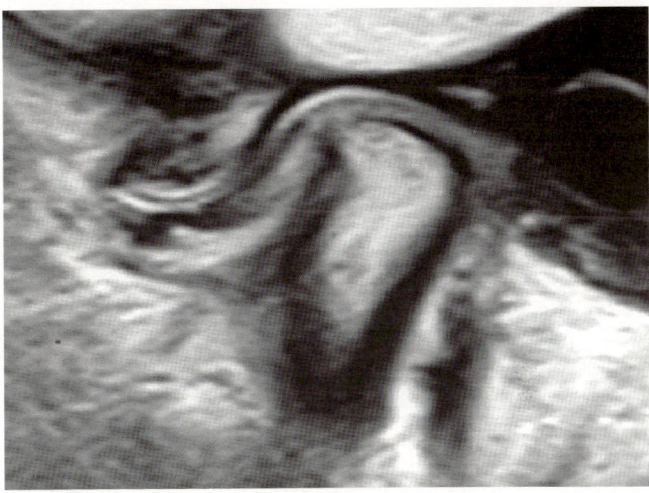

Fig. 8.12: MRI showing disc elongation deformation and increased signal intensity in a case with anterior disc displacement without reduction (ADDWR)

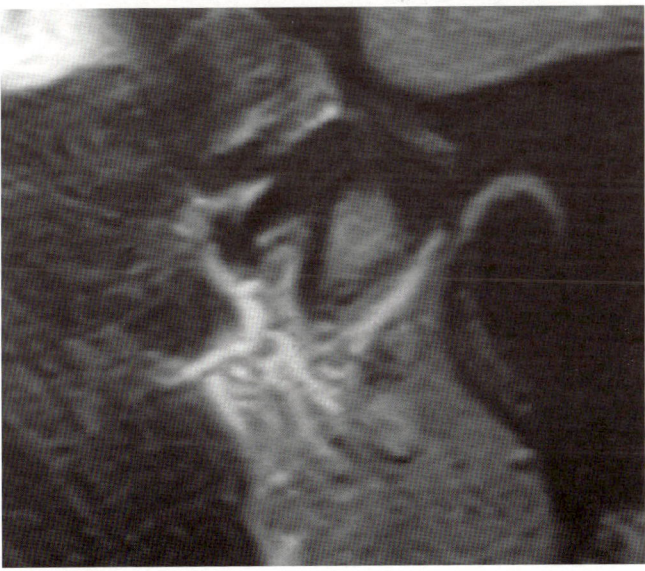

Fig. 8.13: MRI showing thickened posterior band in a case with anterior disc displacement with reduction (ADDR)

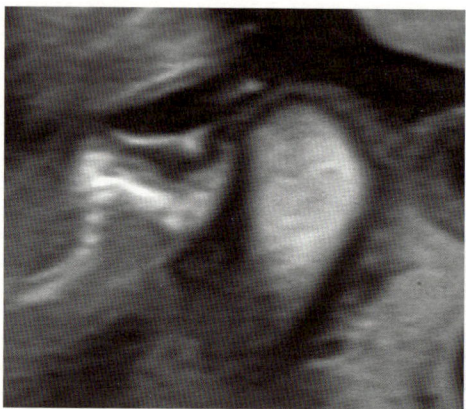

Fig. 8.14: MRI showing flexion deformity, decreased signal intensity and scar tissue in a case with anterior disc displacement without reduction (ADDWR) (open mouth)

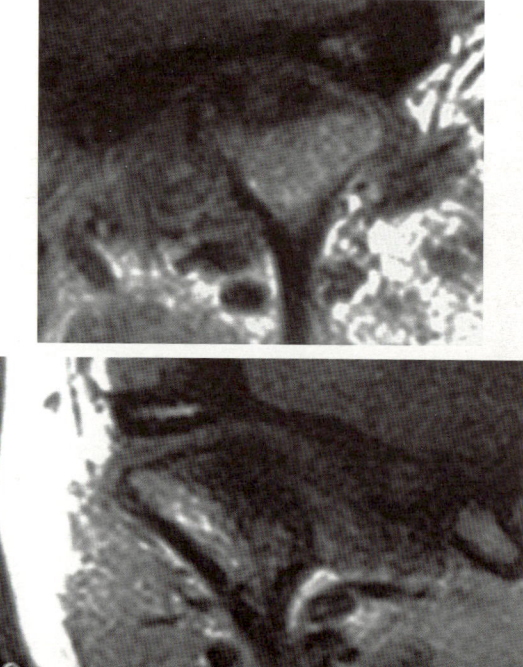

Fig. 8.15: MRI showing osteonecrosis in two cases with anterior disc displacement without reduction (ADDWR)

marrow edema may predict the presence of TMJ pain. An MRI diagnosis of OA was defined by the presence of flattening associated with subchondral sclerosis, surface irregularities and erosion of the condyle or presence of condylar deformities

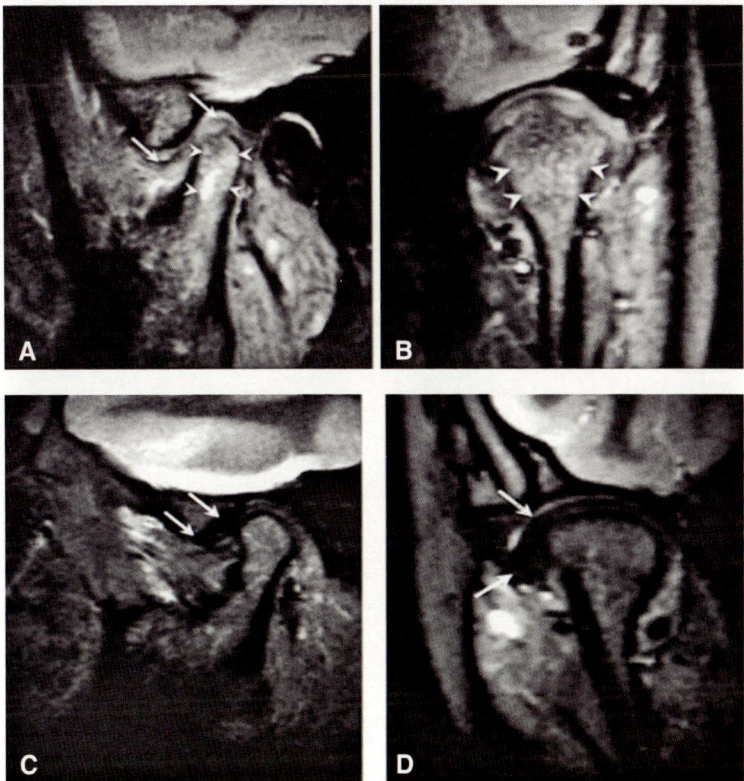

Figs 8.16A to D: Bilateral closed-mouth-related magnetic resonance, or MR, images in a subject with left-side-related temporomandibular joint, or TMJ, pain. (A–B) Left TMJ with presence of disk displacement, or DD; osteoarthrosis, or OA; and bone marrow edema. (A) Sagittal MR image shows disk displaced anteriorly and fragmented (arrows), condyle with flattening and erosion and hyperintensity in bone marrow (arrowheads), indicating the edema pattern, (B) coronal MR image shows condyle with flattening and erosion and increased signal from bone marrow (arrowheads), indicating the edema pattern, (C and D) right TMJ with presence of anterolateral DD and absence of OA and bone marrow edema, (C) sagittal MR image shows disk (arrows) anterior to condyle, (D) coronal MR image showing lateral DD (arrows)

associated with flattening, subchondral sclerosis, surface irregularities, erosion and osteophyte (Fig. 8.16). However they concluded that using magnetic resonance imaging to make diagnoses may not be considered the unique or dominant factor in defining temporomandibular joint disorder populations. Therapy for patients with TMJ based on the evaluation of concomitant morphological abnormalities, whether prophylactically or as treatment for TMJ disorders, may be unwarranted.

Takahashi et al studied the relationship between the presence of joint effusion, joint pain, and protein levels in joint lavage fluid (JL) of patients with internal derangement (ID) and osteoarthritis (OA) of the temporomandibular joint (TMJ). Thirty-eight joints in 26 patients with ID and OA of the TMJ were studied. Magnetic resonance imaging (MRP) evidence of joint effusion was evaluated in T2-weighted images. Samples of JL were collected from the superior joint space during pumping manipulation, and the protein concentration was measured. The presence of pain was based on joint tenderness or a complaint of pain in the preauricular region during mouth opening or closing.

They demonstrated that painful joints are more likely to show joint effusion on MRI, and the protein levels in JL recovered from these joints is higher than in pain-free joints. These data also suggested that joint effusion may be related to the inflammatory changes seen in patients with ID and OA.

Segami et al in 2001 used T2 weighted MR images to detect the relation of joint effusion in TMJ to presence of synovitis. Joint effusion (JE), detected by T2-weighted magnetic resonance imaging (MRI), is prevalent in 30 to 80% of temporo-mandibular joint (TMJ) disorders. JE is believed to reflect intra-articular pathosis; however, to our knowledge, no study has linked the presence of JE, detected by MRI, with direct observations of the inside of the TMJ.

They conclude that, T2-weighted MRI can be a highly clinically significant and useful diagnostic tool for predicting the existence of synovitis—in its ability to detect JE. Our finding that there is a strong relationship between JE and arthroscopic synovitis may help to resolve the clinical puzzle of whether JE is really a sign of synovitis.

Again in 2002 Segami et al conducted another study using T2 weighted images saying that the synovial fluid in joints with joint effusion, shown in T2 images, contain higher protein concentration and the proinflammatory cytokine IL-6, IL-8, than does the synovial in the TMJ without JE.

N Guler et al conducted a study to determine any association between the protein concentration in the synovial fluid and (i) the amount of articular hydrops, as graded in MR images, and (ii) joint pain in TMJs with and without displacement of the disc.

T2 weighted spin-echo images provide information on joint effusion, and inflammatory changes in posterior disk attachment. The form of the disc was also recorded as being normal or showing signs of deformation. On T2 weighted images, joint effusion was identified as an area of high signal intensity in the region of the upper and lower joint spaces. Grading system for categorizing the amount of TMJ fluid on MR images was used as described by Larheim et al (Table 8.1). Joint effusion (JE) may be related to joint pain and inflammatory changes in TMJ with intra-articular disorders. The synovial fluid of a normal joint is not observed on a T2 weighted image because it forms a thin layer. The small amount of synovial fluid in a folded disc collects within the space made by the anterior and posterior band and should be considered a simple case of synovial fluid collection, especially in the painless joint. It is caused by a decrease in positive pressure and by joint effusion. JE has also been observed in asymptomatic joints without clinical symptoms. They conclude that pain in the TMJ

Table 8.1: Grading system for categorising the amount of temporo-mandibular joint fluid

Category	Definition
No fluid	No bright T2 signals from joint compartments (Fig. 8.17)
Minimal fluid	Dots or lines of bright T2 signals along articular surfaces (Fig. 8.18)
Moderate fluid	More than the amount of bright T2 signals defined as minimal fluid and less than the amount defined as marked fluid (Fig. 8.19)
Marked fluid	Equal to this amount of bright T2 signals or more (Fig. 8.20)

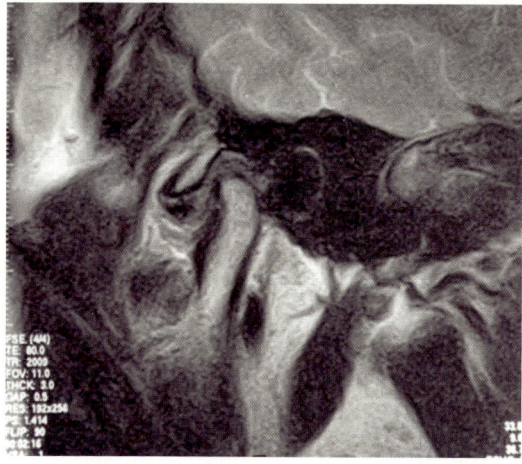

Fig. 8.17: T2 weighted image showing no effusion in the temporomandibular joint

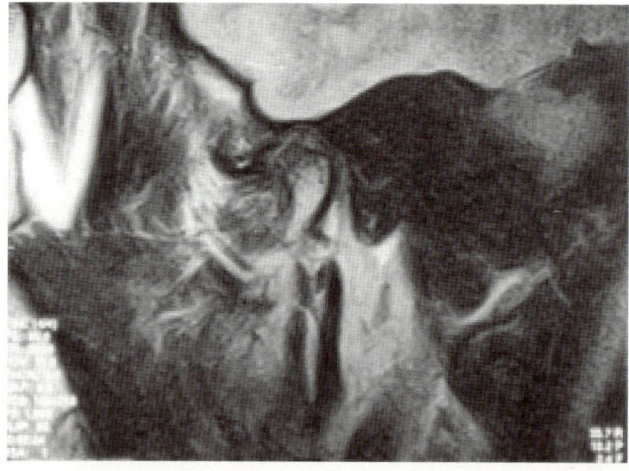

Fig. 8.18: T2 weighted image showing minimal effusion in the temporomandibular joint

was not related to MR findings of JE in internal derangement and synovial fluid aspirate findings of total protein concentration. However, total protein concentration was related to the amount of JE in disc displacement without reduction joints and painful joints were more likely to demonstrate JE.

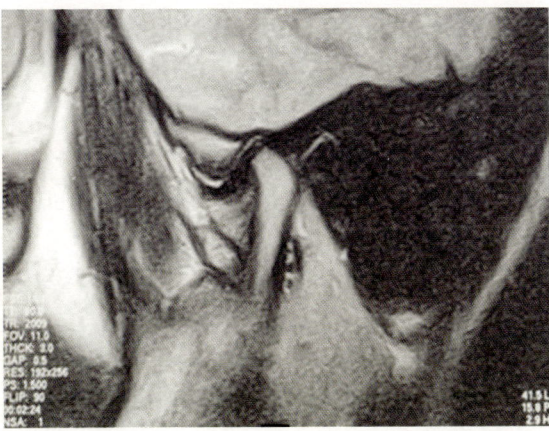

Fig. 8.19: T2 weighted image showing moderate effusion in the temporo-mandibular joint

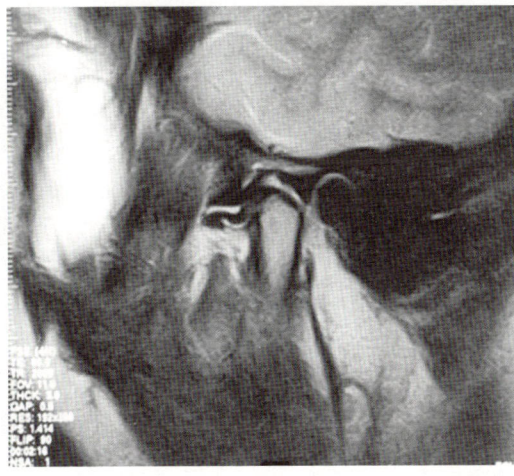

Fig. 8.20: T2 weighted image showing displaced and deformed disc in the lateral part of the temporomandibular joint and marked effusion

BIBLIOGRAPHY

1. Adame CG, Monje F, Offnoz M, Martin-Granizo R. Effusion in magnetic resonance imaging of the temporomandibular joint: a study of 123 joints. J Oral Maxillofac Surg 1998; 56: 314–8.
2. Christiansen EL, Thompson JR. A book on Temporomandibular Joint Imaging. St.Lovie 1990 Mosby pp 147–161.

3. Geva T. Magnetic resonance imaging: historical perspective. J Cardiovasc Magn Reson 2006; 8(4):573–80.

4. Haley DP, et al. The relationship between clinical and MRI findings in patients with unilateral temporomandibular joint pain. JADA 2001; 132:476–81.

5. Katzberg RW, Schenck JF, Roberts D, et al. Magnetic resonance imaging of temporomandibular joint meniscus. Oral Surg Oral Med Oral Pathol 1985;59:3325.

6. Laurel KA, Tootle R, Cunningham R, et al. Magnetic resonance imaging of the temporomandibular joint. II. Comparison with laminagraphic, autopsy and histological findings. J Prosthet dent 1987; 58:211–18.

7. M Schmitter, B Kress, S Hähnel, P Rammelsberg. The effect of quality of temporomandibular joint MR images on interrater agreement. Dentomaxillofacial Radiology 2004;33:253–8.

8. Murakami K, Nishida M, Bessho K, Iizuka T, Tsuda Y, Konishi J. MRI evidence of high signal intensity and temporomandibular arthralgia and relating pain: does the high signal correlate to the pain? Br J Oral Maxillofac Surg 1996; 34: 220–4.

9. N Guler, S Uckan, P Imirzalioglu, S Acikgozoglu. Temporomandibular joint internal derangement: Relationship between joint pain and MR grading of effusion and total protein concentration in the joint fluid. Dentomaxillofac Radiol 2005; 34:175–81.

10. Per-Lennart Westesson Sharon L. Brook. Temporomandibular Joint: Relationship between MR Evidence of Effusion and the Presence of Pain and Disk Displacement AJR 1992; 159: 559–63.

11. Recent development in understanding TMJ disorders. Part II- changes in the retrodiscal tissue. Dentomaxillofac Radiol 2000; 29: 260–3.

12. Rüdiger Emshoff, Iris Brandlmaier, Stefan Gerhard, Heinrich Strobl, Stefan Bertram, Ansgar Rudisch. Magnetic resonance imaging predictors of temporomandibular joint pain. J Am Dent Assoc; 2003:134 (6): 705–14.

13. Sano T, Westesson PL. Magnetic resonance imaging of the temporomandibular joint: increased T2 signal in the retrodiskal tissue of painful joints. Oral Surg Oral Med Oral Pathol Oral Radiol Endod 1995;79:511–6.

14. Sano T, Westesson PL, Larheim TA, Rubin SJ, Tallents RH. Osteoarthritis and abnormal bone marrow of the mandibular condyle. Oral Surg Oral Med Oral Pathol Oral Radiol Endod 1999; 87:243–52. Correction 5, pp 21

15. Segami N, Nishimura M, Kaneyama K, Miyamaru M, Sato J, Murakami KL. Does joint effusion on T2 weighted magnetic

resonance images refect synovitis? Comparison of arthroscopic findings in internal derangements of the temporomandibular joint. Oral Surg Oral Med Oral Pathol Endod 2001;92:341–35.

16. Segami N, Nishimura M, Kaneyama K, Miyamaru M, Sato J, Murakami KL. Does joint effusion on T2 weighted magnetic resonance images refect synovitis? Part 2. comparison of concentration levels of proinflammatory cytokines and total protein in synovial fluid of the temporomandibular joint with internal derangement and osteoarthrosis. Oral Surg Oral Med Oral Pathol Endod 2002;94:515–21.

17. Sharon L Brooks, et al. Imaging of the temporomandibular joint Oral Surg Oral Med Oral Pathol Oral Radiol Endod 1997;83:609–18.

18. S sener, F Akgünlü. MRI characteristics of anterior disc displacement with and without reduction. Dentomaxillofacial Radiology (2004) 33, 245–52.

19. Takahashi T, Nagai H, Seki H, Fukuda M. Relationship between joint effusion, joint pain, and protein levels in joint lavage fluid of patients with internal derangement and osteoarthritis of the temporo-mandibular joint. J Oral Maxillofac Surg 1999;57:1187–93.

20. Westesson PL, Yamamoto M, Sano T, Okano T. Chapter 18: Temporo mandibular joints: anatomy and pathology. In: Som PM, Curtis HD, eds. Head and Neck Imaging. 4th ed. Philadelphia, Pa: Mosby; 2003.

21. White & Pharaoh. Oral Radiology, Principles and interpretation. 5th Edition, pp. 245–64.

22. Yilmaz TN and Toller. A clinical correlation of MRI findings of TMJ; British journal of Oral and Maxillofacial Surgery 2002;40:317–32.

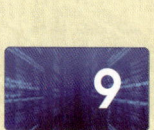

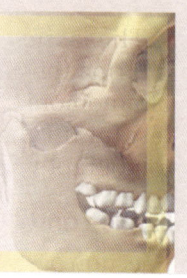

9   TMJ Arthrography

INTRODUCTION

The first successful clinical use of TMJ arthrography to be reported was by Norgaard in the 1947. This procedure basically involved the injection of water-soluble, iodine-containing contrast medium (dye) into the joint space. The procedure is effective and safe but rather technically difficult to do. The technique of Blaschke, Solberg and Sanders involves placing dye in both the superior and inferior joint spaces. It should be noted that fluoroscopy is used to see the correct position of the angiocatheter in relation to the upper and lower joint spaces during insertion. Also, tomography is used after the dye has been placed.

Towards the end of the 1970s several articles appeared, describing the clinical and arthrographic characteristics of internal derangement related to displacement of the disk. These arthrographic studies were actually the first to depict displacement of the disk, a pathologic entity that had been suspected earlier. During the following years, considerable enthusiasm developed for TMJ arthrography, and a large number of publications describing the usefulness of the technique appeared. The changed attitude toward TMJ arthrography can be traced to the following factors:

1. Use of an image intensifier to facilitate joint puncture and to study and document joint dynamics.

2. Identification of disk displacement as a common cause of TMJ pain and dysfunction, and, probably most important

3. Introduction of new, conservative surgical methods for treating disk displacement.

These newer treatment methods required accurate information about the status and function of the joint. The use of a nonionic contrast medium, which made the examination less painful, and the combination of arthrography and tomography, also influenced the increased use of arthrography.

Single- and Double-contrast Arthrography

Injection of contrast medium into only the lower space (Fig. 9.1) is a simplification of the original arthrographic technique, in which contrast medium was injected into both upper and lower joint spaces. This simplification further popularized the use of arthrography; currently, single-contrast lower compartment arthrography is the most commonly used arthrographic technique.

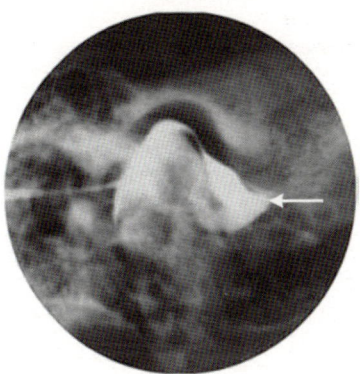

Fig. 9.1: Lower compartment arthrogram of TMJ showing anterior disk displacement. The prominent anterior recess (arrow) of the lower joint space is a sign of disk displacement

Double-contrast arthrography (Fig. 9.2) is a variant of arthrography in which injection of iodine contrast medium is combined with injection of air. The double contrast study is superior to the single-contrast study in its demonstration of the configuration of the disk and the posterior disk attachment (Figs 9.2 and 9.3). However, the double-contrast technique is technically more difficult to perform, because it requires cannulation of both the upper and lower joint spaces and the injection of both contrast medium and air.

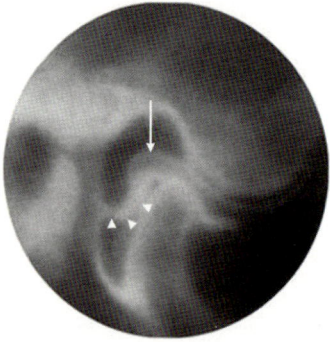

Fig. 9.2: Dual space double-contrast arthrotomogram showing the disk (arrow) in a superior position. The mouth was half open, and the redundant posterior disk attachment (arrow heads) is seen between the disk and the posterior capsule. The upper and lower joint spaces are radiolucent due to the intra-articular injection of air

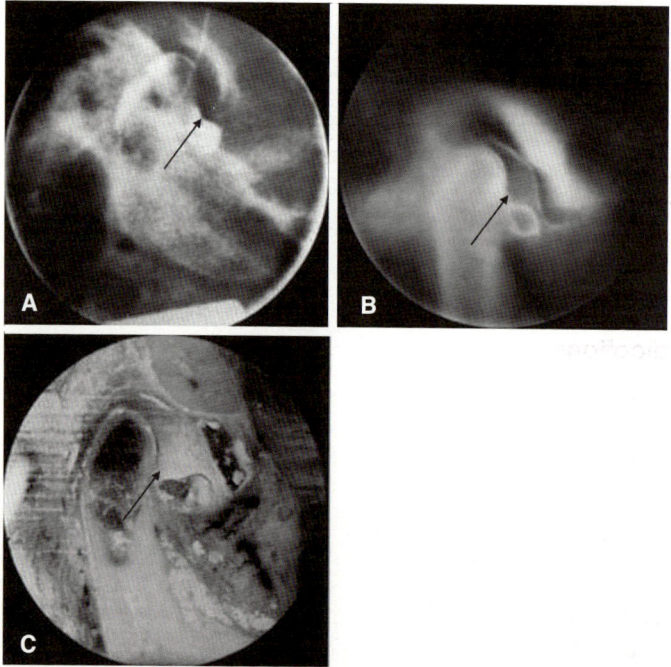

Figs 9.3A to C: (A and B) Single and dual space double-contrast arthrotomography, (C) corresponding cryosection of TMJ with anterior disk displacement. The location of the posterior band is indicated by arrows

Advantages of Arthrography

1. In some instances the soft tissue are a significant part of the disorder, and the injection of a contrast medium helps visualize their shape and position.

2. Through the fluoroscope the clinician can visualize the dynamic movement of the disc and condyle, which may be most helpful in identifying condyle-disc dysfunction.

3. Perforation of the disc can also be visualized with injection of the contrast.

4. Assessment of soft tissue structures of the TMJ

Disadvantages of Arthrography

1. They are somewhat expensive, they are invasive, and they expose the patient to relatively high levels of radiations.

2. The procedure necessitates special training and is not usually accomplished in a general dental office.

3. Injection of contrast medium into the joint spaces causes a ballooning effect of the capsule that tends to separate the articular surfaces.

4. Arthrogram should not be considered as routine radiography for all patients with suspected functionally dislocated disc.

Indications

1. Useful to determine the position, shape, and integrity of the disc and the biomechanics of disc motion as it relates to condylar translation in patients with TMJ dysfunction.

2. Aspiration through the needle placed for arthrography may yield inflammatory fluid, crystals, or purulent material, which can aid in the diagnosis.

3. Arthrography allows accurate determination of the position of the disk and can show joint dynamics.

4. Perforation of the disk can be diagnosed. (But false positives have been reported to occur in as many as 20% of cases).

Contraindications

Contraindication to arthrography includes:

1. Infection of the overlying skin.
2. Prior history to contrast material.
3. Bleeding diathesis or anticoagulant therapy.

PROCEDURAL TECHNIQUE

Anesthesia

For single space arthroscopy, the auricular temporal nerve is anesthetized. With the help of a small bore needle, infiltration of the skin and underlying soft tissues is done with 1% lidocaine. Both the compartments may be entered from a single point of entry on the skin. Five tenth milliliter of 1:1000 epipherine mixed with the 10 ml of isotonic, nonionic contrast material slows the absorption of contrast but does not cause tachycardia and hypertension that may occur with higher concentrations of epinephrine if the contrast is inadvertently injected intravenously.

Entering the Joint

The patient is placed in a supine oblique position with the head lateral and the body of the mandible parallel to the table top. With the mouth in the closed position, the posterior slope of the articular surface of the mandibular condyle is localized fluoroscopically and this point is marked on the overlying skin. The mouth is opened slightly to increase the retromandibular space. After sterile preparation and draping of the preauricular skin, the needle is directed anteriorly to the condyle and walked off its posterior margin into the joint. If a 3 ml or smaller volume syringe (23-gauge needle) is used, there is a noticeable difference in the ease of injection upon entering the joint space. One tenth to two tenth of a milliliter of lidocaine is injected into the joint with reflux back through the needle upon removal of the syringe if the needle tip is intra-articular. Using fluoroscopic guidance, approximately 0.5 ml of contrast material is injected into the posterior recess of the inferior joint space, noting its appearance ventral to the condyle. Occasionally, over distension may cause reduction of a displaced disc by creating tension on the retrodiscal attachment.

The upper joint compartment may be entered through the same injection site in the skin, so additional local anesthetic is not necessary. With the mouth open, the needle is directed cephalad and anteriorly toward the posterior auricular surface of the articular eminence. As with the lower compartment, using a small syringe results in a noticeable difference in the ease of injection upon entering the joint. With the mouth open there frequently is negative pressure in the upper compartment, so care must be taken not to allow air to enter the joint upon removal of the syringe. The surface of glenoid fossa and eminence will be outlined. A larger volume of contrast material (1 to 1.5 ml) is required in the superior space than in the inferior space. Over distention may cause the patient discomfort, both may alter disc function, making it more difficult to assess. The needle length required for most patients is about 2 cm (Figs 9.4 to 9.7)

CONTRAST TECHNIQUE

Single contrast arthrography, the common method, is the filling of the joint compartment with radiopaque contrast medium before radiography. The single contrast technique is usually combined with tomography, improving the radiographic representation of the joint. In double contrast arthrography, the articular surfaces are coated by radiopaque medium and

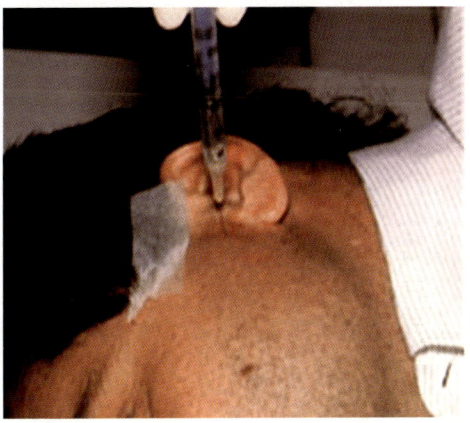

Fig. 9.4: Injection of a contrast medium in arthrography

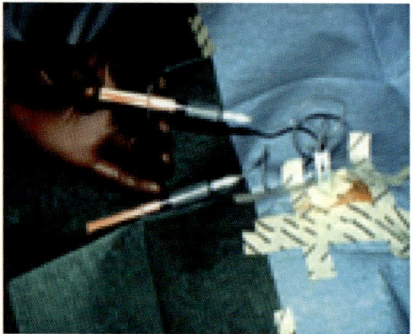

Fig. 9.5: Arthrographic dyes

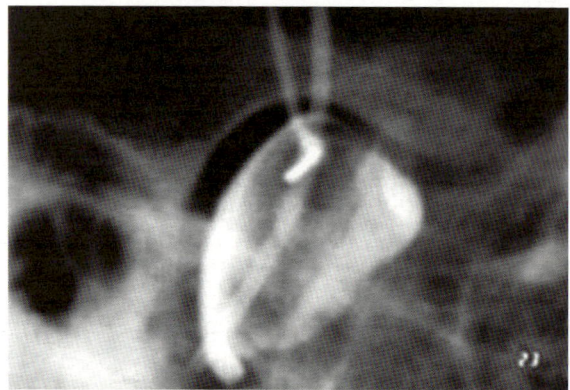

Fig. 9.6: Arthrographic images

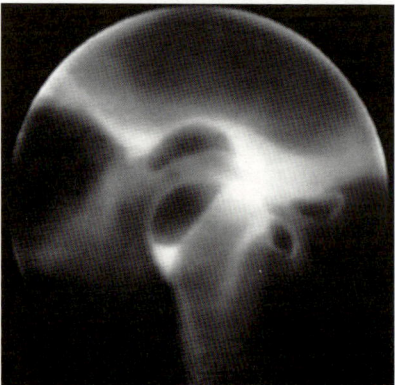

Fig. 9.7: Arthrogram of temporomandibular joint

the joint compartment is expanded by air. Double contrast arthrography has been widely applied to other joints.

Non-ionic contrast agents are less irritating to the synovium and if used in an isotonic dilution they will not lose density through the absorption of water into the joint. It is difficult to keep a contrast medium in the joint for contemplative filming because of rapid absorption by the vascular synovium. Absorption may be retarded by using epinephrine; however its systemic effects must be avoided.

In 1980, Westesson, Omnell and Rohlin modified the technique and reported on dual contrast method of arthrotomography. They suggested that dual contrast method was superior for early recognition of contour abnormalities of the joint cartilage. This also facilitated the diagnosis of internal derangement of the disc complex. The dual contrast is achieved with the combined injection of positive contrast material and air. A comparison study was done in 1984 to determine the correlation of dual contrast arthrotomography with postmortem morphology.

FLUOROSCOPY, CINEFLUOROGRAPHY AND VIDEOFLUOROGRAPHY

Most modern special procedure X-ray units are equipped with a video recorder and freeze frame fluoroscopy. It is therefore no longer necessary to use the high exposure technique of cineradiography to do joint functions studies during arthrography. Considerable patient exposure can be saved by intermittent fluoroscopy for needle placement using freeze-frame viewing.

PLAIN RADIOGRAPHY

Fluoroscopic spot films and plain films result in less radiation exposure to the patient than tomography, and they can be done quickly and easily. However tomography has the advantage of blurring superimposed osseous and soft tissue shadows. For documenting disc position and pattern of movement, video fluorography and spot films may be adequate when using single-compartment, inferior space arthroscopy. It may be necessary to supplement the study with tomography when superimposition of structures poses a problem. Dual compartment arthrography, which gives better detail of disc morphology and joint surface features, is not optimally performed without tomography. Coronal images may be necessary when the disc appears normally positioned but thinned, yet jaw opening is impaired. Coronal projections show lateral and medial disc displacements.

TOMOGRAPHY

The finest image detail is obtained with thin section tomography. The disadvantage which lies in this technique is that it takes time to perform multiple, closely spaced sections through the joint in closed and open jaw positions and unless the procedure is done with skill contrast may be lost from the joint before the study is completed. Three to four thin sections in the closed position and one or two sections in the open position may prove adequate if properly located. The coronal views should be corrected for condylar angulation to be most effective for showing mediolateral components of displacement. The disadvantage of increased radiation exposure, which occurs with arthrotomography, is because of the need for multiplanar views.

COMPUTED TOMOGRAPHY ASSISTED ARTHROGRAPHY

Computed tomography assisted arthrography is better than arthrotomography for showing the details of disc position and morphology. The disadvantage with this technique is that in coordinating the two portions of the procedure. If the CT scan is not done promptly after injection of the joint, contrast material is lost from the joint and the images do not clearly show the disc features. A second disadvantage is the time required for image multi formatting after the scanning.

NORMAL ARTHROGRAM

Inferior Compartment

Temporomandibular joint arthrograms are conventionally viewed in the sagittal plane. Coronal projections are supplementary. The opacified inferior compartment caps the condyle with a slightly bulbous ventral recess in the closed mouth position. The ventral cephalad margin of the ventral recess may be either flat or concave depending on the shape of the adjacent ventral band of the disc. The dorsal space extends well down onto the neck of the condyle and is bounded caudally by the retrodiscal attachment. When the jaw opens, contrast material is squeezed from the ventral space into the dorsal space, but because of the tension on the inferior band of the retrodiscal attachment and the rigidity of the posterior discal band, the dorsal space becomes tented toward the junction of the posterior band and its attachment.

During hinging and translation with opening, the condyle and disc move as a unit with a smooth progression of the condyle, which comes to rest ventral to the summit of the articular eminence. The corrected coronal projection reveals a crescent of contrast material conforming to the shape of the condyle and the underside of the disc.

Dual Compartment

In the closed mouth position, contrast material in the superior compartments conforms to the articular surface of the glenoid fossa and articular eminence. The dorsal limit of the superior compartment is at the petrotympanic fissure, the insertion of the retrodiscal attachment. The ventral recess of the superior compartment extends beneath the articular eminence, where it may have a slightly bulbous appearance. In the corrected coronal plane, the opacified superior compartment forms a double crescent above the disc with lateral and medial recesses approximating the lateral and medial recesses of the inferior compartment. With progressive jaw opening, the dorsal recess of the superior compartment widens and becomes bulbous with a flattened convex curve toward the retrodiscal attachment. With both compartments opacified, the interposed disc is outlined by the contrast material. The pattern is characteristically that of an eccentric biconcave lens with the thicker portion superior to the condyle. With the mouth open, the central thinner part of the disc resides between the eminence and the condyle.

ABNORMAL ARTHROGRAM
Discal Perforation

Fluoroscopy is important for diagnosing perforations of the disc. If a hole in the retrodiscal attachment or the disc itself is large, contrast material appears in the superior compartment early during the injection. If the contrast medium appears late, the perforation is probably small, limiting the flow, or the needle position may have changed, penetrating the discal attachment. Occasionally, the jaw opening and closing are necessary to demonstrate communication. When contrast appears first in the superior space, one must suspect that the superior compartment has been entered directly or through the lower compartment, perforating the retrodiscal attachment.

DISC DISPLACEMENT WITH REDUCTION

Displacement of the disk with reduction (Fig. 9.8) and without reduction (Fig. 9.9) are the most frequent pathologic findings in TMJ arthrography. Principally this means that the posterior

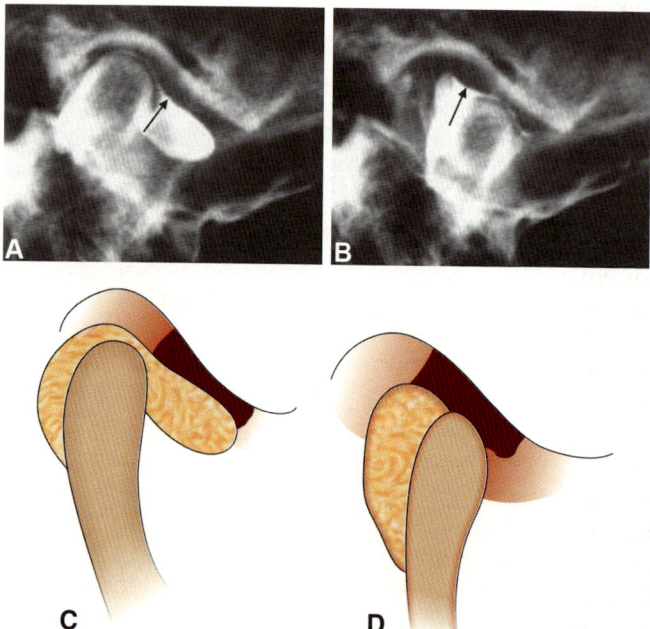

Figs 9.8A to D: (A and C) Anterior disk displacement demonstrated with single-contrast lower compartment arthrography. The posterior band (arrow) of the disk is located anterior to the condyle, (B and D) after reduction the disk is in a normal superior position with the posterior band (arrow) posterior to the condyle

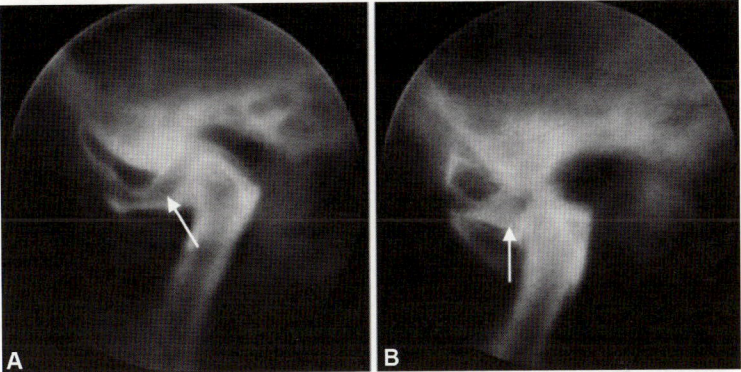

Figs 9.9A and B: Anterior disk displacement without reduction, double-contrast arthrogram. (A and B) with closed mouth and maximum mouth opening, the disk is located anterior to the condyle. The position of the posterior band is indicated by arrows

thick part (posterior band) of the disk is located anterior to the condyle in the closed-mouth position, and the condyle closes on the posterior disk attachment (bilaminar zone). An arthrographic sign of disk displacement in single-contrast lower compartment arthrography is enlargement of the anterior recess of the lower joint space. In disk displacement with reduction the disk is usually biconcave, although there may be some minor enlargement of the posterior band. This corresponds to the early intermediate stage in the classification scheme described by Wilkes. In disk displacement without reduction a more extensive deformity of the disk is frequently encountered, and this corresponds to the late stage in the same classification scheme. This is consistent with the deformities observed in pathologic specimens, which include thickening and shortening of the anteroposterior dimension of the disk. Perforation of the posterior disk attachment is another sign of late-stage internal derangement. Perforation is indicated by passage of contrast medium from the lower to the upper joint space (Fig. 9.10) when only the inferior space is injected.

Altered disc function is associated with laxity of the discal attachments. The disc loses its close attachments to the condyle, with resultant redundancy of the medial, lateral and posterior attachments. This may suddenly as with trauma in which the capsule is stretched or torn, or it may develop slowly. Defects

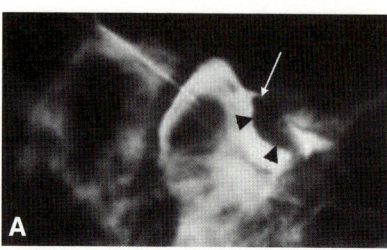
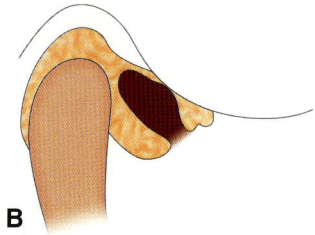

Figs 9.10A and B: Perforation. (A) Contrast material was injected into the lower joint space, and there is an overflow (arrow) to the upper joint space indicating perforation. The disk (arrowheads) is anteriorly displaced and deformed, (B) schematic drawing of A

on the joint fibrocartilage surface may cause obstruction along the path of disc movement resulting in asynchronous disc and condylar function. When the ligaments of the joint are worn out, the disc tends to become displaced either medially, laterally, anteriorly or posteriorly. The most common disc displacement is anteriorly and anteromedially.

Depending on the degree of disc displacement, the condition of attachment and the joint surfaces, the disc may come back to its normal position during some phase of the open-close cycle. When this occurs, the disc usually comes back rapidly to its normal position resulting in a popping or clicking sound. The term "reciprocal clicking" is used to designate the noises associated with the disc first as it moves onto the condyle during jaw opening and second as it moves off the condyle during jaw closing.

Arthrography in the closed mouth position shows a concave impression on the cephalad aspect of the enlarged ventral recess of the inferior joint compartment, caused by the thickened posterior band of the ventrally displaced disc. Just before disc reduction during opening, the contrast material becomes partly squeezed from the bulbous ventral recess. With reduction, the ventral recess thins to normal as the condyle negotiates the articular eminence. During jaw closing as the disc again becomes displaced, the widened ventral recess is reformed.

Dual compartment studies show widening of the ventral recess of the superior compartment until the disc is reduced as well. This results from the buckling of the disc which causes the ventral recess to gape. With contrast in both compartments, the outline of the misshapen disc profile usually is discernible as well.

DISPLACEMENT WITHOUT REDUCTION (CLOSED LOCK)

The displaced disc may not return back to its normal relationship with the condyle when jaw opening is attempted. This condition is called closed lock. In cases of chronic disc displacement the jaw may open normally even though the disc remains displaced. Chronic discal changes such as these are frequently accompanied by acquired bony changes in the joint, mainly the condylar component and perforation of the disc or its posterior attachment. The arthrogram typically shows restricted translation as the result of limited opening. The widened ventral space of the inferior compartment is maintained throughout the restricted open close cycle. With dual compartment opacification, the ventral recess of the superior compartment remains dilated and the shape of the disc usually distorted, is evident.

Since a chronically dislocated disc usually has an altered shape, dual compartment arthrography often reflects the shape of the disc. Most commonly the disc becomes folded in the cephalad direction so that it produces a concave contour along the cephalad margin of the ventral recess. Occasionally a disc may appear thinned in its sagittal profile on the dual compartment opacification, but the patient may have restricted opening and pain. Sideways and rotational displacement should be suspected in this situation and coronal tomograms should be obtained.

Westesson et al described the variation in the normal temporomandibular joint arthrographic anatomy. According to them a small anterior recess of the lower joint compartment has been considered a sign of normal disc position, whereas a large or medium-size recess has been considered a sign of disc displacement. A convex or flat upper margin of the anterior recess of the lower joint compartment has been considered as an indicator of a superior disc position; whereas a concave upper margin has been looked upon as a sign of disc displacement.

JOINT BODIES

Loose bodies impair joint function in the temporomandibular joint just as in any other synovial joint. Usually the cause of these loose bodies is not known, although they are sometimes caused by osteochondritis disscans. These loose bodies result in osteochondral bodies or joint mice, which may be difficult to visualize within the joint compartment during arthrography.

ADHESIVE CAPSULITIS

As a result of inflammation, the joint compartment and their recesses may contract, and the condition is known as adhesive capsulitis. The common causes of inflammation include hemarthrosis, usually from trauma. Nonspecific inflammation may occur idiopathic or with autoimmune disorders.

Less commonly, pyarthrosis may occur as result of infection caused by organisms such as *Neisseria gonorrhoeae*, *Salmonella*, *Staphylococcus*, and *Streptococcus*. Adhesions form, binding opposing joint surfaces, restricting movement of the condyle, retracting the disc and producing pain. Introducing a needle in such a joint is challenging.

POSTOPERATIVE ARTHROGRAMS

Postoperative changes in the joint appear to be related to the type of surgical procedure. Westesson and Ericksson did double contrast arthrotomography in 10 patients who had been treated by diskectomy 1–3 years earlier. Difficulty was encountered in injecting the small joint space in one patient, who subsequently was shown to have extensive intra-articular adhesions. The remaining nine patients had reasonably good joint function.

Bronstein also reported on the results of postoperative arthrography in patients undergoing retrodiscal transactions and repair. Four studies were non-diagnostic and eight showed a pattern of capping of the condyle with adhesions. The author concluded that postoperative arthrography cannot be considered useful as an indicator of surgical success. Both CT and MRI have been used along with arthrography for studying patients after surgery for complications of permanent prosthetic disc implants made of laminates of Proplast and Teflon. Arthrography does not seem to offer any advantage for postoperative follow-up of these patients.

DIAGNOSTIC ACCURACY

Generally the accuracy of arthrography has been directed towards its ability to diagnose disc displacement, perforations or other internal derangements. Using operative findings, arthrography's accuracy has been reported to be 81 to 97%. Westesson and Rohlin reported a diagnostic accuracy of 85% for their technique of double contrast arthrotomography using cryosectioning of the cadaver joints for correlation. Single air contrast arthrography was tried for the first time in 1988 by Ohnishi et al. Further, Honda et al recently reported application of single air contrast arthrography along with limited cone beam computed tomography for diagnosis of temporo-mandibular joint disorders in patients allergic to iodine. They reported a case of a patient visiting the hospital with TMJ pain and difficulty of mouth opening. As she had claustrophobia and could not tolerate iodine, they elected to perform air contrast arthrography and pumping manipulation therapy. The air contrast arthrography showed that the articular disk was slightly anteriorly displaced, the disk configuration was biconcave, and an adhesion as well as a perforation of the disk was present. The result of the examination was effective for diagnosis.

Westesson studied double contrast tomography of the temporomandibular joint, he conclude in his study that double contrast arthrotomography demonstrate clearly the intra-articular anatomy of TMJ and produces useful information for treatment planning. The arthrographic diagnosis essential when conservative treatment has failed and the desirability of surgical intervention for repair or excision of the disc is being considered. GC Anderson et al evaluate the reliability of clinicians in predicting an arthrographic diagnosis of articular disc position in a typical patient population presenting for TMJ arthrographic evaluation. Two clinicians utilized a brief history, clinical examination (including evaluation of mandibular movement and TMJ auscultation), and tomographic TMJ imaging in evaluating 60 patients. The radiologist subsequently performed the arthrographic procedures on 102 TMJs (18 unilateral and 42 bilateral). Diagnostic agreement was determined for all possible diagnostic categories including: normal disc position, TMJ internal derangement with reduction,

TMJ internal derangement without reduction/acute, TMJ internal derangement without reduction/chronic, and osteoarthrosis. The significance of the diagnostic agreement between the clinicians and arthrography was evaluated with a Kappa Statistical Test, which showed good reliability.

The future of arthrography depends on the establishment of proven treatment methods for disc displacement and progress toward improved resolution of MRI.

BIBLIOGRAPHY

1. Blaschke, DD, Solberg, WK, Sanders, B. Arthrography of temporomandibular joint: review of current status, J.Am. Dent. Assoc.100:388, 1980.
2. Book on common disorders of temporomandibular joint, Chapter 4 Radiographic Evaluation by James V. Manzione page no. 40–61.
3. Christiansen EL, Thompson JR. A book on Temporomandibular Joint Imaging. St.Lovie 1990 Mosby.
4. Clyde A. Helms and Phoebe Kaplan Diagnostic Imaging of the Temporomandibular Joint: Recommendations for Use of the Various Techniques. AJR: 154,319–322 Feb 1990.
5. GC Anderson, EL Schiffman, KP Schellhas, JR Fricton. Clinical vs. Arthrographic Diagnosis of TMJ Internal Derangement. J Dent Res 68(5):826–829, May, 1989.
6. Honda K, Matumoto K, Kashima M, Takano Y, Kawashima S, Arai Y. Single air contrast arthrography for temporomandibular joint disorders using limited cone beam computed tomography for dental use. Dentomaxillofacial Radiology 2004; 33: 271–3.
7. Jeffery P Okeson. Management of Temporomandibular Disorders and Occlusions pp 3–28
8. Norgaard, F. Arthrography of mandibular joint, Acta Radiol 1944,25:679.
9. Uysal S, Kansu H, Akhan O, Kansu O. Comparison of ultrasonography with magnetic resonance imaging in the diagnosis of temporomandibular joint internal derangements: a preliminary investigation. Oral Surg Oral Med Oral Pathol Oral Radiol Endod 2002;94(1):115–21.
10. Westesson PL, Omnell KA, Rohlin M. Double contrast tomography of the temporomandibular joint: a new technique based on autopsy specimen examination. Acta Radiol Diag 1980;21 (6) 777–84.
11. Westesson PL, Rohlin M. Diagnostic accuracy of double contrast arthrotomography of the temporomandibular joint: correlation with postmortem morphology. Am J Neuroradiol 1984;54;463–8.

12. Westesson PL. Diskectomy of the temporomandibular joint: a double contrast arthrotomographic follow-up study. Oral surg Oral med Oral pathol 1985;59:435–40.
13. Westesson PL, Ericsson L, Kurita K, Malmo and Lund. Temporo-mandibular joint: Variation of normal arthrographic anatomy. Oral Surg Oral Med Oral Pathol 1990;69:514–9.
14. Westesson PL, Yamamoto M, Sano T, Okano T. Chapter 18: Temporomandibular joints: anatomy and pathology. In: Som PM, Curtis HD, eds. Head and Neck Imaging. 4th ed. Philadelphia, Pa: Mosby;2003.

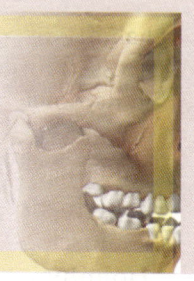

10   TMJ Arthroscopy

INTRODUCTION

Arthroscopy is a technique of introducing an optical instrument into the joint allowing direct visual examination of its internal surfaces. Dentists frequently see patients with pain and clicking of the TMJ, tenderness of muscles of mastication, and limitation of jaw opening. Conservative treatment with counselling, jaw exercises, muscle relaxants, splint therapy, occlusal equilibration, or a combination of the above are then used. However, the presence of intracapsular pathology and gross displacement of the disc preclude a response to conservative therapy only. Arthroscopy has been introduced as a diagnostic, and recently, as a therapeutic tool which may eliminate the necessity for some patients to have open TMJ surgery.

HISTORY AND DEVELOPMENT

Endoscopy in orthopaedic surgery was first attempted by Takagi in 1918 using a cystoscope to examine a knee joint. With the advances in the technology of fiberoptic light systems; knee joint arthroscopy became popular in orthopaedic surgery. It was not until 1974 when Ohnishi initiated the first application of arthroscopy to TMJ. The technology is available in Hong Kong and the Department of Oral Surgery and Oral Medicine has been using the arthroscope for 2 years. Ohnishi was the first to describe the application of arthroscopy to the TMJ. He, along with Murakami and Kino, defined the terminology, pathology, and anatomy of TMJ arthroscopy.

The development of smaller arthroscope and surgical proficiency provided data for studies that confirmed the reliability of arthroscopy. Moses and Poker suggest that the success of arthroscopy may be attributed to–

1. Removal of inflammatory substances by lavage.
2. Increased disc mobility.
3. Reduced adverse loading of supporting joint structures
4. Reduction of synovial inflammation as a possible cause of muscle strain and fatigue.

Holmlund & Helsing in 1985 in a study of 54 cadavers evaluated the diagnostic accuracy of 2 different arthroscopes a rod lens system and a so called Selfoc system. The upper joint compartment was found to be punctured with accuracy and without damage to vital tissues.

Advantages

1. Arthroscopic observations of TMJ provide a direct, detailed look at the actual surfaces of the joint and the disk, which cannot be obtained with other diagnostic methods.
2. The improved visualization of joint structures can be recorded on videotape and retrieved for documentation and future reference.
3. The procedure can be accomplished in 10 to 30 minutes in which diagnosis and lavage are completed through a small incision or puncture that does not always require suturing.
4. Jaw mobilization is immediate after arthroscopy with full range of motion resumed within 3 days. In most cases, patients can resume daily activities within 3 days.
5. The cost of arthroscopy is consistently lower than that of arthrotomy.
6. Arthroscopy can also be used to confirm the position of the articular disc before proceeding with orthodontic therapy and disc position can be correlated with the final tooth positioning.
7. It is very effective in resolving pain and improving function in patients with non-reducing discs.

Disadvantages

1. It is a invasive procedure.
2. Special training and equipment is required.

3. Complications although rare are potentially more serious, for example, middle ear perforation.

4. Arthroscopy does not permit meticulous manipulation and suturing of malpositioned disc.

ARTHROSCOPY TECHNIQUE

Patient Selection

Patients with signs and symptoms of intracapsular disorders such as disc displacement, hypomobility, osteoarthritis, and synovitis with adhesive capsulitis; unresponsive for at least 3 months of conservative therapy are candidates for TMJ arthroscopy. Arthroscopy is usually performed on an outpatient basis but under general anesthesia. Nasoendotracheal intubation is preferred. A preauricular approach is preferred and the patient is prepared and the surgical field sterilized. The patient's mouth is draped with steridrapes to allow the surgeon's assistant to manipulate the mandible.

Various techniques and entry points have been reported, although most surgeons agree that the arthroscope should be inserted slightly anterior to the tragus of the ear in line with the lateral canthus of the eye along the Langer's lines.

A 21 gauge needle attached to a 10 ml syringe filled with normal saline is inserted into the glenoid fossa from a point near the tragus of the ear and is directed anteriorly, superiorly and medially. Once the glenoid fossa is entered, 3–5 ml of normal saline is injected to expand the superior joint space. The down ward and forward hydraulic displacement of the condyle is noted by the assistant surgeon. After the needle is removed, a 2–4 mm vertical entry incision is made anterior to the tragus. A sharp trochar is placed through the arthroscopic canula and inserted in the same pathway as the needle that carried the normal saline. After the lateral capsule is pierced with the trochar, care is taken not to insert it further to avoid disruption of the joint relationships. A uniflow efflux needle is directed 5 mm anterior to the arthroscopic cannula, and lavaging the joint with normal saline confirms the location. An outflow needle deposits the effluent into a calibrated receptacle. This system permits the lavage volume to be controlled, preventing extravasations of the irrigating fluid into surrounding tissues. The irrigation solution provides for expansion of the superior joint space so that examination and repair procedures can be accomplished more easily. It is also used to remove debris and provide a clear field of view. It reduces the probability of intracapsular sepsis.

A 0 degree wide angle 10- or 15-degree arthroscope is selected for the diagnostic phase of the procedure. The arthroscope is attached to a fiberoptic light source that is coupled to a video camera. A TV monitor is used for viewing that enlarges the field of view compared to viewing directly into the lens of the arthroscope. The fiberoptic bundles in the arthroscope illuminate the joint cavity, and the procedure is documented on videotape. Newer technology permits video printing that can be done in the operating room and that has improved lines of resolution and subsequent image clarity.

Examination begins in the superior joint recess (orienting to the 12 o'clock position) by noting the integrity of the retrodiscal tissues. Then the position of the disc and the inclination of the articular eminence is noted. Care is taken not to disrupt the fibrocartilage covering the articular eminence so that adhesions or surface erosions can be documented. The assistant then manipulates the mandible so that the relationship of the articular disc to the mandibular condyle is noted.

Then the anterosuperior recess is examined. In many instances this recess is restricted and the covering of the articular eminence is torn. Restriction of the articular recess may be mistakenly thought to arise from discal adhesions, when they are primarily caused by restriction of the lateral ligament. Entrance to the anterior recess is best gained either laterally or medially with the jaw in a semiclosed position. The location, size, and shape of the articular disc are registered as its attachment to the lateral pterygoid muscle.

After the examination, the joint is thoroughly lavaged, and the incision is closed with fine suture. Corticosteroids are injected into the capsule in cases with inflammatory or degenerative disease. Intraoral occlusal splints are inserted immediately after examination.

Arthroscopic surgery is done after joint examination except in cases where restrictive fibrosis prevents initial viewing. In such cases fibrotic lesions are lysed by blind blunt trochar sweeps before arthroscopic viewing. A vertical incision is positioned 20 to 30 mm anterior and 10 mm inferior to a line drawn from the lateral canthus of the eye to the tragus of the ear. The 30 degree arthroscope is preferred for panoramic viewing and for the visualization of working instruments. It is advantageous to use an arthroscopic sheath for the working cannula should it be necessary to obtain different views of the joint. Appropriate rubber stoppers have been developed to allow the interchange of diagnostic and working cannulas.

COMPLICATION

1. As with all surgical procedures, there are risks involved. Fortunately, the risks and complications from TMJ arthroscopy are few and minor, but can be potentially serious.
2. Bleeding from the superficial temporal vessels is not uncommon due to the close anatomical path to the joint.
3. When anatomical landmarks are mistaken, neurological damage to the auriculotemporal nerve or the facial nerve can occur.
4. Scuffing of the Intracapsular surfaces can easily happen if care is not taken with the sharp trocar.
5. Extravasations of irrigation fluid into the surrounding tissues occurs with overzealous irrigation, although it is readily reversible and poses only a minor complication.
6. Severe complications are rare and include:
   - Seventh cranial nerve damage
   - Middle ear damage
   - Blood vessel lysis
   - Perforation of middle cranial fossa
   - Holmlund and Hellsing reported a low incidence of insult to the facial nerve and superficial temporal artery.

ARTHROSCOPIC ANATOMY

Synovial Membrane and Retrodiscal Tissue

The synovium lines the inner capsular surface as a translucent membrane with its greatest concentration in the retrodiscal tissues. Laterally and medially, the joint capsule blends with the retrodiscal tissues but is less vascular. As the retrodiscal tissues extend posteriorly, their vascularity diminishes as they attach to the glenoid fossa. Anteriorly, the retrodiscal tissues join with the avascular disc. This sharply demarcated junction should be easily observed in a normal joint but is often absent in cases of disc degeneration.

When the condyle is positioned superiorly within the glenoid fossa, the retrodiscal tissues may blanch and should not be mistaken for the articular disc. During condylar translation the elastic retrodiscal tissues should maintain a smooth appearance on their surface.

ARTICULAR DISC

The smooth, white, textured, biconvex superior surface of the disc blends medially and laterally with the capsule and anteiorly with the superior belly of the lateral pterygoid muscle. In the normal joint the thick posterior discal band lies over the superior crest of the condylar process.

The intermediate zone appears where the condyle meets the articular eminence and rotates over the eminence during translation. The anterior discal band resides in the anterior recess, and in some cases the three regions of the disc can be observed when the condyle is deflected inferiorly.

ARTICULAR EMINENCE

Variations in the shape and steepness of the articular eminence are common. The inferior margin of the eminence may range from relatively flat to sharply concave. Normally, the steepness is approximately 45 degrees. During arthroscopic access to the anterior recess, the fibrocartilage covering the eminence is usually minimally disrupted unless there is joint hypermobility.

ANTERIOR RECESS

To gain access to the anterior recess, the condyle should be deflected inferiorly but not anteriorly. Then, with the jaw partially open, the arthroscope is advanced slowly. In cases where there is restriction of the anterior recess, a 30 degree arthroscope is used to give a more panoramic field of vision. The superior belly of the lateral pterygoid muscle is easily identified by its color (bluish in most normal joints) and striations as it attaches to the disc and the anterior eminence.

INFERIOR JOINT SPACE

Usually examination of the inferior joint space is not necessary. However, in cases of disc perforation or osteoarthritis, it can be helpful. The articular fibrocartilage covering the condyle has a glistening white appearance in the normal joint. Small irregularities in the surface of the fibrocartilage are common and do not indicate a pathologic condition. Synovial folds are fewer than in the superior joint compartment, and the demarcation between disc and peridiscal tissues is less distinct. The posterior band of the disc flows smoothly into its retrodiscal attachment.

PATHOSIS

Inflammatory Changes or Synovitis

Increased vascularity in localized areas was noticed with capillary hyperemia, as reported in the arthroscopy based synovitis index of Holmlund and Hellsing.

SYN 0: Normal pale, almost translucent, synovial lining with a fine network of anastomosing small blood vessels.

SYN I: Localized area with increased vascularity and capillary hyperemia, contact bleeding may occur during arthroscopy.

SYN II: Generalized capillary hyperemia, effusion and debris. Arthroscopic examination is possible after irrigation of the joint cavity.

DISC DISPLACEMENT

Trauma and abnormal joint relationships may cause disc to become displaced. In symptomatic patient, disc displacement is more common anteriorly than laterally and medially. As a result of prolong stretching, the retrodiscal tissues lose their elasticity, become redundant and show surface irregularities. Also, the disc loses its gloss and changes shape. In prolong disc displacement the synovium does not penetrate the articular surfaces and there is a tendency for chondromalacia. The roughened surface of the fibrocartilage will adhere to inflamed tissue, leading to adhesions and joint fibrosis. It is possible that joint hypomobility from disc displacement is a greater contributor to painful joint than the disc-condyle relationship.

Blaustein et al described the five diagnostic markers of disc displacement:

1. The presence of remodelled retrodiscal tissue: a dull, white tissue with a variable number of surface vessels interposed between normal retrodiscal tissue and posterior band (remodelled).
2. The remodelled retrodiscal tissue is topographically related to the medial capsular ligament.
3. A flexure is created by the junction of a pink, vertically oriented tissue (retrodiscal tissue) with a horizontally oriented white tissue with surface vascularity (remodelled retrodiscal tissue).
4. In the dynamic examination phase, the condyle contacts remodelled retrodiscal tissue.
5. In the posteriorly fields, the joint space is funnel shaped.

PERFORATION

Initial retrodiscal perforations appear with frayed margins, where as long-standings have rounded, rolled, smooth margins. Subsequent surface osteoarthritis (loss of the articular cartilage) may be the result of inflammatory and proteoglycan by–products rather than actual mechanical abrasion. With perforation, joint sounds usually are grinding or coarse crepitus in nature. Depending on the location of the perforation mechanical open–locking is possible. Once the perforation enlarges to a point where the disc no longer impinges between the condyle and the glenoid fossa, pain seems to lessen for most patients.

ARTHROSIS

Chronic displacement of the articular disc may lead to changes in disc morphology and function with out perforation. Fibrillations and fibrous adhesions produce diminished surface viscosity, which in turn leads to hypomobility. Restriction of the joint space with osseous remodelling makes examination difficult. it may become necessary to lyse adhesions to permit arthroscopy. This group of patients has the poorest response to arthroscopy, and arthrotomy should be considered earlier in the treatment.

ADHESIONS

Adhesions are more permanent and are caused by a fibrosis attachment of the articular surfaces. When adhesions are permanent, the disc function can be great. When adhesions are present breaking the fibrous attachment is the only definite treatment. This can often be achieved with arthroscopic surgery. The surgery breaks up adhesions, and the lavage used to irrigate the joint during the procedure assists in decreasing symptoms. Murakami et al reported on a comparison between the clinical signs and symptoms and severity and distribution of the adhesions. The results indicate that although adhesions might alter the joint mobility, they contribute little to TMJ pain and dysfunction.

Arthroscopy appears to be more sensitive in the identification of the remodelled retrodiscal tissue. The operator can detect subtle changes in the surface of these tissues that are not apparent during gross examination. Arthroscopy offers the clinician the opportunity to enter the joint and to examine under direct vision the affected tissues. The procedure permits this examination without attendant sequelae of an open procedure and in considerably less time.

BIBLIOGRAPHY

1. Blaustein David, et al. Diagnostic Arthroscopy of the Temporomandibular joint Oral Surg Oral Med Oral Pathol 1988; 65 (2) 135–41.
2. Cheung LK, et al. Current advances in TMJ Arthroscopy 1990:39–41.
3. Chilvarquer I, Freitas A, Glass BJ, Chilvarquer LW, et al. Intercondylar dimension as a positioning factor for panoramic images of the temporomandibular region. Oral Surg Oral Med Oral Pathol 1987; 64:768–73.
4. Christiansen EL, Thompson JR. A book on Temporomandibular Joint Imaging. St.Lovie 1990 Mosby.
5. Holmund A, Hellsing G. Arthroscopy of the temporomandibular joint. An autopsy study. Int J Oral Surg 1985; 14(2): 169–75.
6. Holmlund A, Hellsing G. Arthroscopy of the TMJ: Occurrence and location of osteoarthrosis and synovitis in a patient material. Int J Oral Maxillofac Surg 1988; 17: 36–40.
7. Murakami K, Segami N, Moriyay, Itzuka T. Correlation between pain and synovitis in patients with internal derangement of the TMJ. J Oral Maxillofac Surg 1992;50:705–78.
8. Ohnishi M Arthroscopy of the Temporomandibular joint; J Stomatol Soc Jpn 1975; 42:207–13.

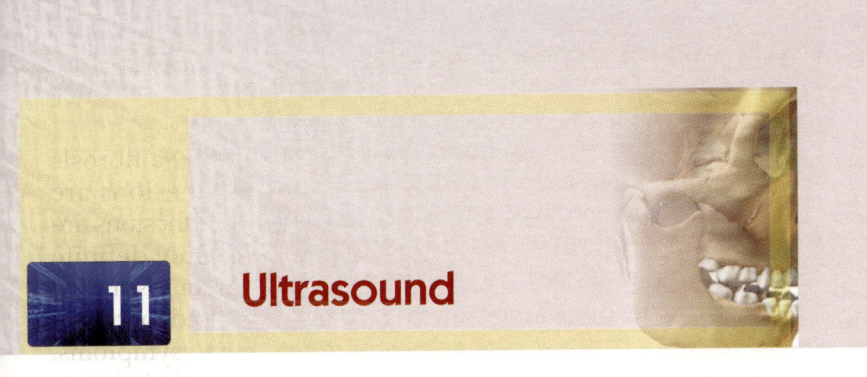

11 Ultrasound

Temporomandibular joint ultrasonography is a non-invasive, readily available and relatively cheap dynamic "real time" examination, featuring soft joint tissues. It serves both for diagnosis and differential diagnosis and for the comparison of therapeutic results in treating internal joint defects. The first reports of TMJ sonography date back to 2000. It uses currently available types of ultrasonic equipment with a linear scanning transducer of 7.5–12 MHz frequency, which makes it possible to depict the narrow space of the jaw joint and the position of the joint disc and it reveals fluid or ligament adhesion. During the examination, the patient is in the sitting position and the transducer is placed on the skin above the joint parallel to the long axis of the mandible branch. The joint disc is scanned on the screen as a thin homogen hypo, as far as the isoechogen strip contiguous to the condyle border. The condyle bone borders and articular eminence show as a hyperechogen line. During the examination it is possible to directly observe the joint disc move when the mouth is opening and closing. Studies comparing the results of MRI and sonography showed 70–85% agreement. An ultrasonographic system using the high frequency and conveyors with a large diameter has been recently invented. The ultrasonograph waves, generated by this system, are able to penetrate easily through the small aperture between the glenoid fossa and the condyle. This new ring transducer has a high focus depth and narrow wave beam. The bone surface rebounds as much as 2/3rds of the waves, only 1/3rd propagating down to deeper structures. For this reason the transmitter must be placed on a specific place, with the aim to transmit waves through the soft tissues, situated between the condyle and the eminence.

The principle of ultrasonography is based on the fact that ultrasonic sound waves emitted by a device (transducer), travel through the tissue against which they are aimed, and are partly reflected on transiting through dissimilar anatomical structures. The reflected sound waves are then read by the same emitting device, and translated into images.

Diagnostic ultrasonography (sonography), the clinical application of ultrasound, uses vibratory frequencies in the range of 1 to 20 MHz. Scanners used for sonography generate electrical impulses that are converted in to ultra-high-frequency sound wave by a transducer, a device that can convert one form of energy into another – in this case electrical energy into sonic energy. The most important component of the transducer is a thin piezoelectric crystal or material made up of a great number of dipoles arranged in a geometric pattern. A dipole may be thought of as a distorted molecule that appears to have a positive charge on one end and a negative charge on the other. Currently, the most widely used piezoelectric material is lead zirconate titanate (PZT). The electrical impulse generated by the scanner causes the dipoles in the crystals realign themselves with the electrical fields and thus suddenly change the crystal's thickness. This abrupt change begins a series of vibrations that produce the sound waves that are transmitted in to the tissues being examined.

As the ultrasonic beam passes through or interacts with tissues of different acoustic impedance, it is attenuated by a combination of absorption, reflection, refraction and diffusion. Sonic waves that are reflected back (echoed) towards the transducer cause a change in the thickness of the piezoelectric crystals, which in turn produces an electrical signal that is amplified, processed and ultimately displayed as an image on a monitor. In this system the transducer serves as both a transmitter and a receiver. Current techniques permit echoes to be processed at a sufficiently rapid rate to allow perceptions of motions; this is referred to as real time imaging.

In contrast to X-ray imaging, in which the image is produced by transmitted radiation, the reflected portion of the beam produces the image in sonography. The fraction of the beam that is reflected back to the transducer depends on the acoustic impedance of the tissue, which is a product of its density (and thus the velocity of sound through it) and the beam's angle of incidence. Because of its acoustic impedance, a tissue has a characteristic internal echo pattern. Consequently, not only can changes in echo patterns delineate different tissues, but they also can be correlated with pathologic changes in a tissue.

ULTRASOUND AND TEMPOROMANDIBULAR JOINT

Ultrasound uses a transducer that functions as a transmitter and a receiver of acoustic energy. Ultrasounds emitted by the transducer are partly reflected when they pass through the tissues, with a coefficient of reflection that depends on the characteristics of different anatomical structures (e.g. cortical bone has the highest echogenicity, which reflects most of the ultrasound waves; soft tissues have a lower echogenicity). The same transducer receives the reflected ultrasounds, translating them into images.

The TMJ area, which includes bone (condylar and temporal bone), connective (joint capsule and rertrodiscal tissues), fibrocartilaginous (disk), and muscular (lateral pterygoid and masseter muscles) tissues, has some peculiarities with respect to other musculoskeletal areas. The small examination area, with limited accessibility to the deep structures, and the high risk of ultrasound reflecting off bone tissues make the interpretation of images complex. The imaging protocol includes transverse and longitudinal scans so the antero-superior joint compartment can be examined in coronal, axial and oblique views. A linear probe, with a frequency of 7.5–20 MHz is placed over the TMJ, perpendicular to the zygomatic arch and parallel to the mandibular ramus and tilted until the best view is achieved. When a satisfactory view is obtained, static and dynamic evaluations are usually performed at different mouth opening positions.

Cortical bone tissues, such as the head of the condyle and the glenoid fossa, are generally hyperechoic (high reflection of sound waves) (Figs 11.1 and 11.2); appearing white on US images, while bone marrow is usually hypoechoic (low reflection of sound waves) and appears black. Connective (joint capsule and retrodiscal area) and muscular tissues (lateral pterygoid and masseter muscles) are isoechoic (intermediate reflection of sound waves) and appear heterogeneously grey

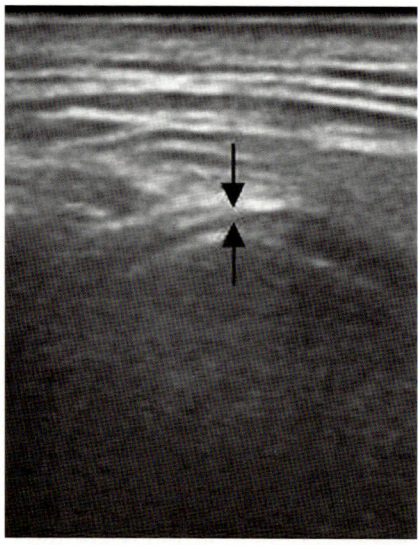

Fig. 11.1: US of the TMJ. Hyperechoic lines (white) represent the glenoid fossa (superior line) and condylar surface (inferior line), respectively. The distance between the two lines is an indirect measure of joint effusion due to capsular distension. Surface irregularities may suggest the presence of bone remodelling

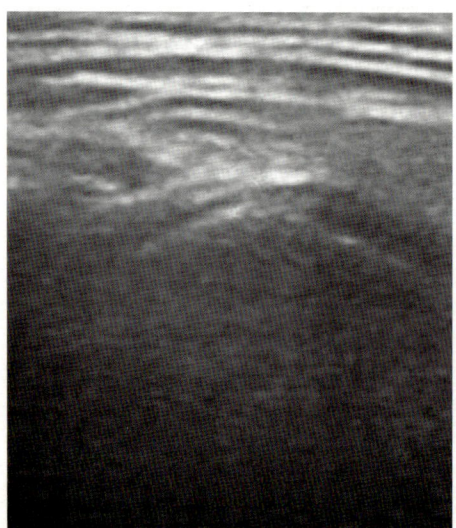

Fig. 11.2: US image of an oversized TMJ condyle

in US images. Empty spaces and water (superior and inferior joint spaces) are hypoechoic (black), even though they are virtual cavities that are usually not detectable, unless effusion is present.

Motoyoshi M et al described a way of positioning the transducer that would allow a better visualization of the head of the condyle and the disc that are usually hidden by the temporal bone. The authors suggested rotating the transducer 60 degrees from the horizontal plane, following the plane of the articular eminence, and tilting it 5–10 degrees from the line perpendicular to the sagittal plane in order to have access from above the zygomatic process of the temporal bone.

Landes et al suggested the use of ultrasonography for measurement of mandibular range of motion obtaining 83% agreement with axiographic results. They also reached values of sensitivity, specificity and accuracy close to 90% for the diagnosis of disc displacement with reduction (DDWR), compared to MRI, using both horizontal and vertical positioning of the transducer (Figs 11.3A and B).

Magnetic resonance imaging (MRI) has been considered the most accurate method for visualizing the disc-condyle relationship and to confirm the clinical suspicion of disc displacement. Its accuracy is about 95% when sagittal and coronal scans are evaluated. The main disadvantages of MRI are non-availability in some centers, high cost and restricted use in patients with claustrophobia, cardiac pacemakers and metallic prostheses. In the last decade, ultrasonography (US) has been used as a new method for diagnosing TMJ disc displacement, with the advantages of being noninvasive and less expensive than any other imaging technique used with this goal.

Disk Position and Morphology

Elias MF et al conducted a study in which joints free of disc displacement underwent ultrasonographic evaluation in order to identify some standards of normality, which could be used in future studies as indirect signs to assess the disc position. Ultrasonographic investigation was accomplished with longitudinal and transverse scans in the closed- and open-mouth positions, with the transducer overlying the TMJ and

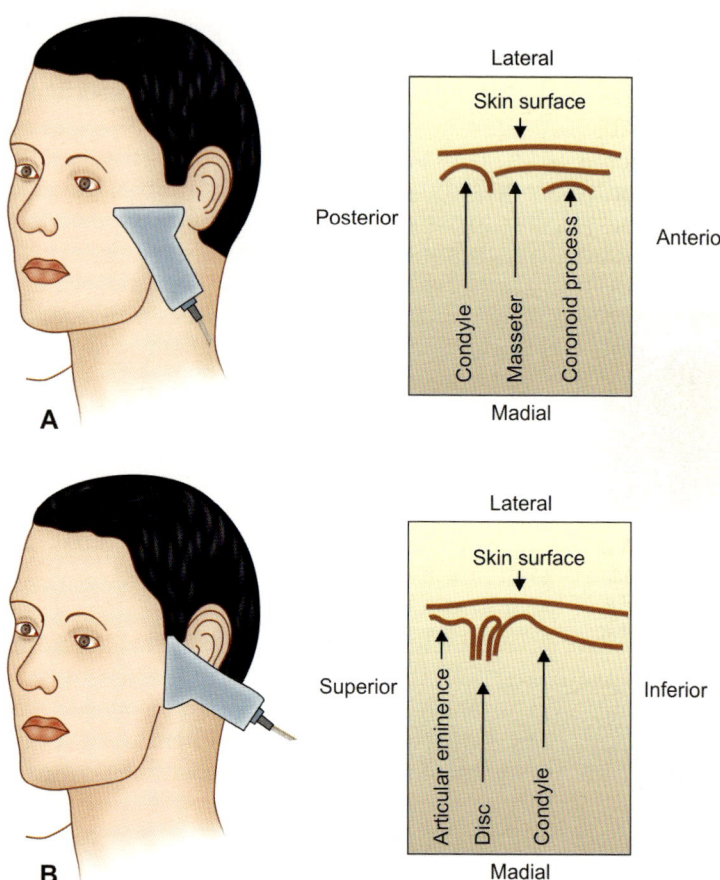

Figs 11.3A and B: Positioning of the transducer and consequent visualization of the temporomandibular joint (TMJ). (A) Horizontal positioning, transverse image of the TMJ, (B) Vertical positioning, coronal/sagittal image of the TMJ (depending on the angulation of the transducer)

the zygomatic arch. Tilting the transducer over its long axis was necessary to obtain optimal visualization of the articular structures. The scanning was performed by the same radiologist and repeated 3 times for each closed- and open-mouth position, while all the images were being recorded. In each scan, the operator measured the distance between the most lateral point of the articular capsule and the most lateral point of the mandibular condyle (lateral capsule-condyle distance).

Afterwards, the distance between the most anterior point of the articular capsule and the most anterior point of the mandibular condyle (anterior capsule-condyle distance) was measured. When visible, a normally positioned disc could be identified as an echogenic structure surrounded by a hyperechogenic line, corresponding to the articular capsule (Fig. 11.4).

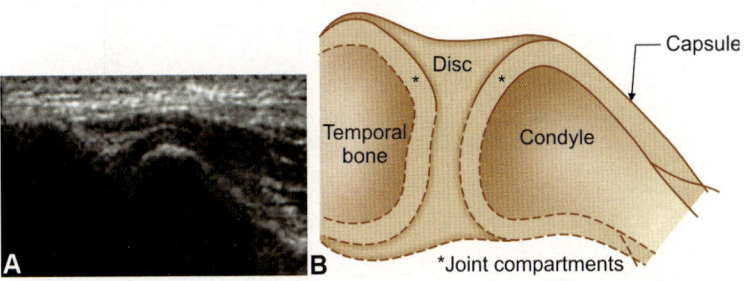

Figs 11.4A and B: Longitudinal (coronal) ultrasonographic scan of the TMJ (A). In the diagram (B), the broken lines correspond to the structures that are not able to be visualized. The top of the figure is guided to lateral and the left to superior

Because of inconstant visualization of the disc in all sonograms, lateral and anterior capsule-condyle distances were used as indirect ultrasonographic signs to determine disc position, since these distances could be measured in all the exams (Figs 11.5 to 11.8).

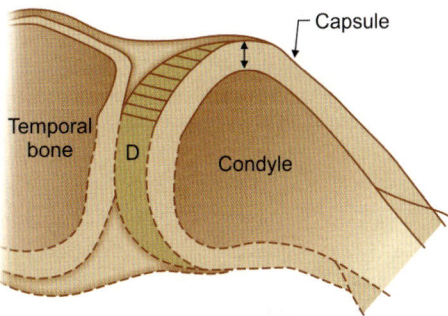

Fig. 11.5: Diagram of a longitudinal (coronal) ultrasonographic scan of the TMJ, showing the lateral capsule-condyle distance (double-ended arrow). The broken lines correspond to the structures which are not able to be visualized (D = disc)

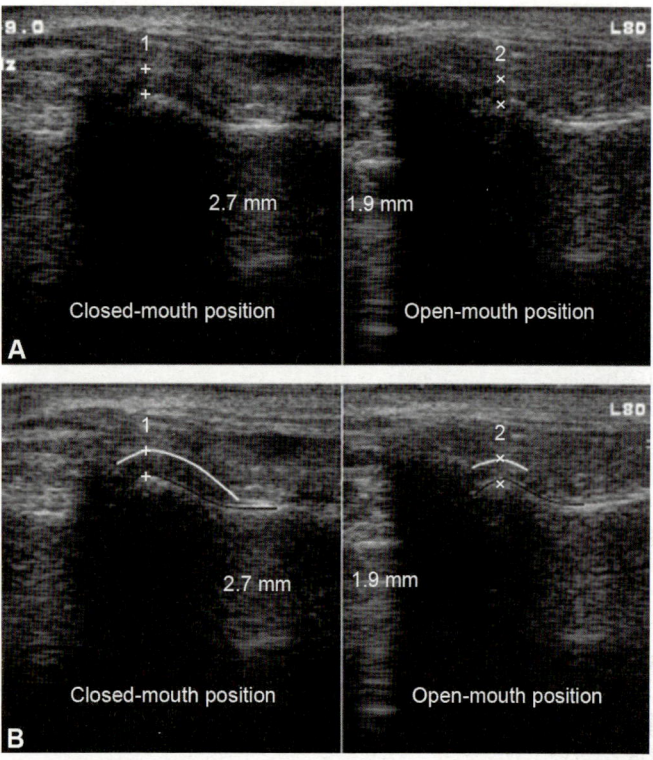

Figs 11.6A and B: (A) Lateral capsule-condyle distance, as seen in a longitudinal (coronal) ultrasonographic scan, in the closed-mouth position (1 = 2.7 mm) and open-mouth position (2 = 1.9 mm). The top of the figure is guided to lateral and the left side to superior. (B) Same image shown in (A), with the contour of the capsule and condyle

Elias MF et al concluded that the measurement of the distance between the most lateral point of the articular capsule and the most lateral point of the mandibular condyle (lateral capsule-condyle distance) can be used to assess the lateral position of the disc, whereas the measurement of the distance between the most anterior point of the TMJ capsule and the most anterior point of the mandibular condyle (anterior capsule-condyle distance) can be used to assess the anterior position of the disc.

A recent report by Jank et al reported accuracy of 92% and 90% with closed and open mouth positions, respectively, with a sensitivity of 86–92% and a specificity of 91–92%.

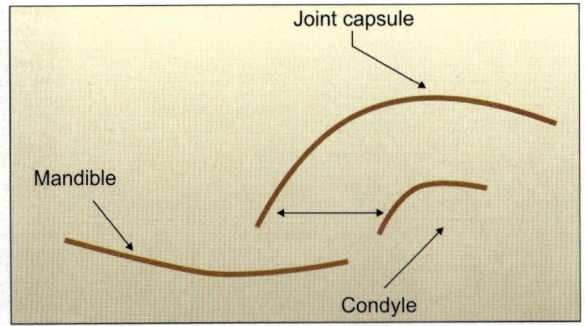

Fig. 11.7: Diagram of a transverse (axial) ultrasonographic scan of the TMJ, showing the anterior capsule-condyle distance (double-ended arrow). The top of the figure is guided to lateral and the left side to anterior.

Emshoff R et al assessed the value of ultrasonography as a diagnostic aid in patients with TMDs. This study included 17 patients presenting with signs and symptoms of TMD. To determine the diagnostic value of static and dynamic ultrasonography in detecting the presence or absence of disk displacement at various mouth opening positions, subjects underwent clinical, ultrasonographic, and MRI investigation. Ultrasonographic investigation using longitudinal to transverse scans was performed with a linear (B-scan) 7.5 MHz small-part transducer. The transducer was connected to a Picker (Picker International GmbH, Vienna, Austria) echocamera (CS 9300), with the diagnosis made directly from the screen. They reported a low sensitivity of the procedure, but a high specificity, especially in the dynamic evaluation (95–100%). They concluded that dynamic ultrasonography is an inexpensive and noninvasive diagnostic technique with relatively high specificity that could be used to supplement clinical evaluation in patients with TMJ disorders. It may help in the identification of normal disk position in subjects presenting with signs and symptoms of TMJ internal derangements.

JOINT EFFUSION

Ultrasound has been widely employed to detect effusion in many musculoskeletal areas; it is accurate at depicting the presence of intra-articular inflammatory fluids in larger joints.

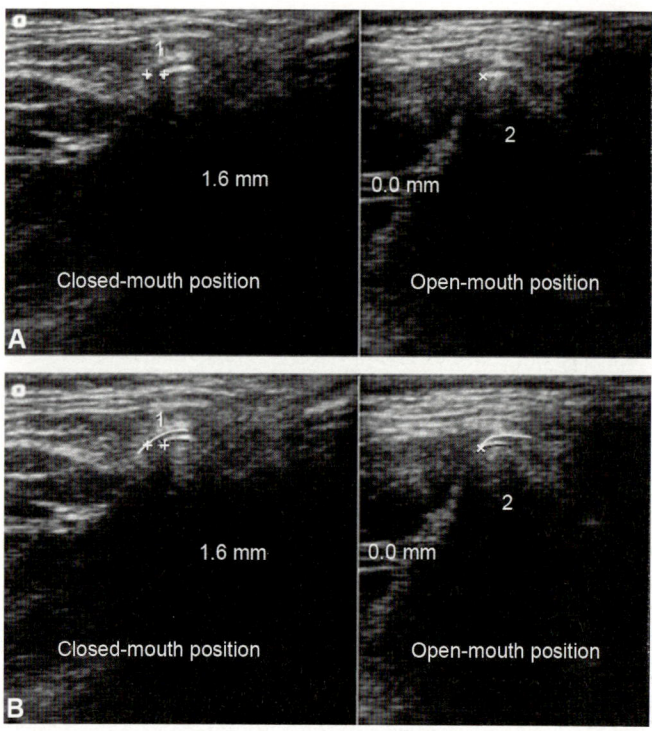

Figs 11.8A and B: (A) Anterior capsule-condyle distance in a transverse (axial) ultrasonographic scan, in the closed-mouth (1 = 1.6 mm) and open-mouth (2 = 0.0 mm) positions. The top of the figure is guided to lateral and the left side to anterior. (B) Same image shown in (A), with the contour of the capsule and condyle

TMJ effusion, as depicted with imaging techniques, is likely to be related to clinical pain on palpation, which appears to be related to images of joint effusion and not disk position abnormalities. A preliminary study by Manfredini et al reported good agreement (80%) between a US diagnosis of joint effusion and clinical pain on joint palpation. There is consensus that the presence of joint effusion may be detected by direct visualization of a hypoechoic area within the articular space or by an indirect measurement of capsular distension, taken as the distance between condylar laterosuperior surface and the articular capsule (a hyperechoic line running parallel to the surface of the mandibular condyle) with the subject in the closed-mouth position (Fig. 11.9).

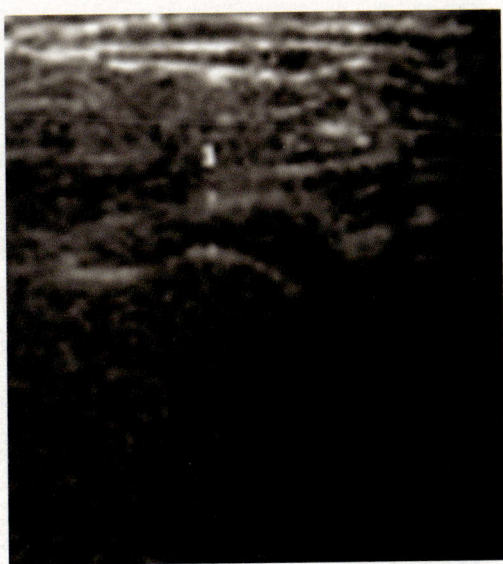

Fig. 11.9: The presence of joint effusion can be detected indirectly by measuring the distance between the two articular surfaces (clips)

Data on the TMJ came from studies assessing the presence of abnormalities within the condylar surface, which are often referred to as osteoarthrosis. US diagnosis of erosions is commonly based on the detection of an interruption or absence of the echogeneity of the cortical lining. Owing to the deflection of sound waves by bone structures, the medial aspect of the condyle can hardly be depicted, and osteophyte formation and condylar erosion are more easily seen in the anterior or lateral aspect of the condyle. Condylar morphology is best seen on longitudinal scans, but transverse investigation may help to increase the examiner's confidence that the condyle has osteoarthrosis.

BIBLIOGRAPHY

1. D Manfredini, L Guarda-Nardini. Ultrasonography of the temporo-mandibular joint: a literature review. Int. J. Oral Maxillofac. Surg. 2009;38:1229–36.

2. Elias FM, Birman EG, Matsuda CK, Oliveira IRS, Jorge WA. Ultrasonographic findings in normal temporomandibular joints. Braz Oral Res 2006;20(1):25–32.
3. Emshoff R, Bertram S, Rudisch A, Gassner R. The diagnostic value of ultrasonography to determine the temporomandibular joint disk position. Oral Surg Oral Med Oral Path 1997;84:688–96.
4. Landes C, Walendzik H, Klein C. Sonography of the temporo-mandibular joint from 60 examinations and comparison with MRI and axiography. JCraniomaxillofac Surg 2000;28:352–61.
5. Melis M, Secci S, Ceneviz C. Use of ultrasonography for the diagnosis of temporomandibular joint disorders: A review. American Journal of Dentistry, Vol. 20, No. 2, April, 2007;73–8.
6. Tvrdy P. Methods of imaging in the diagnosis of temporomandibular joint disorders. Biomed Pap Med Fac Univ Palacky Olomouc Czech Repub 2007, 151(1):133–6.
7. White, Stewart C., Pharoah, Michael J Oral radiology Principles and Interpretation 5th edition **Published by** Mosby. pp 262–3.

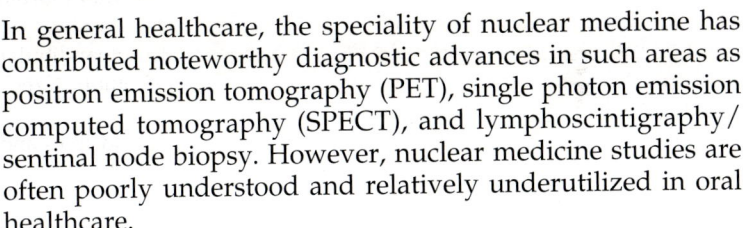

12   Nuclear Medicine

In general healthcare, the speciality of nuclear medicine has contributed noteworthy diagnostic advances in such areas as positron emission tomography (PET), single photon emission computed tomography (SPECT), and lymphoscintigraphy/ sentinal node biopsy. However, nuclear medicine studies are often poorly understood and relatively underutilized in oral healthcare.

Film radiography, CT, MRI, and diagnostic ultrasonography are considered morphologic imaging techniques; that is, each requires some specific structural difference or anatomic change for information recorded by an image receptor. In film radiography, for example, perception of an image depends on contrast, which in turn partly depends on the differential absorption of X-rays. The dependence of X-ray imaging on differential absorption essentially limits this technique to a single variable (tissue electron density), which in turn is presented as a structural or anatomic difference. However, human disease can exist with no specific anatomic changes. Changes that are seen may simply be later effects of some biochemical process that remains undetected until physical symptoms develop. Radionuclide imaging (or functional imaging) provides the only means of assessing physiologic change that is a direct result of biochemical alteration.

Radionuclide imaging is based on the radiotracer method, which assumes that radioactive atoms or molecules in an organism behave in a manner identical to that of their stable counterparts because they are chemically indistinguishable. Radiotracers allow measurement of tissue function *in vivo* and provide an early marker of disease through measurement of biochemical change. Radionuclide-labelled tracers are used in

159

quantities well below amounts that are lethal to cells. However, in spite of the fact that radionuclide imaging is considered noninvasive, the radiation dose the patient receives as a result of intravenous injection of radionuclide-labelled tracers should be considered. It has been reported that injection of $3.7X \times 10^8$Bq of ^{99m}Tc-pertechnetate delivers a whole–body radiation dose of 1 mGy. This quantity is about one third the average annual effective doses resulting from natural radiation. Although many gamma-emitting isotopes have been used in radionuclide imaging, including iodine (^{131}I), gallium (^{67}Ga), & selenium (^{74}Se), the one most commonly used is technetium 99m (^{99m}Tc). As technetium pertechnetate, ^{99m}Tc mimics iodine distribution when injected intravenously. Additionally, when it is manipulated chemically and attached to other compounds, it can be used to perform scans of virtually every organ of the body.

The use of tracers for diagnostic imaging became possible with the development of, first, the rectilinear scanner and, later, the Anger or gamma scintillation camera. Both these instruments record the gamma emissions from patients injected with appropriate tracers. The cameras use a scintillation crystal that has the ability to fluoresce on interaction with gamma rays. This flash of light (fluorescence) is detected by a photomultiplier tube that magnifies and amplifies the signal. The amplified signal is digitized and ultimately used to produce an image by computer algorithm. Use of a scintillation crystal for acquisition of data for image formation has led to the labelling of this technique as scintigraphy. A stationary Anger camera or a rectilinear scanner is capable of producing a flat-plain image of an area or organ in question.

Use of an Anger camera with the capacity to rotate 360 degrees about the patient or specialized ring detectors makes single photon emission computed tomography (SPECT) possible.

In this technique, either multiple detectors or a single moving detector allows acquisition of data from a number of contiguous trans-axial slices, similar to CT by X-ray. These data can be used to construct multiplanar images of the area of study. An even more recent development than SPECT in the field of nuclear medicine is positron emission computed tomography (PET).

PET, which is reported to have sensitivity nearly 100 times that of a gamma camera, relies on positron-emitting radionuclides generated in a cyclotron.

After injection of the radionuclide in to the patient, the isotope with in the body's tissue emits a positron. This positron then interacts with a free electron and mutual annihilation occurs, resulting in the production of two 551 keV photons emitted as 180 degree to each other. When electronically coupled opposing detectors simultaneously identify this pair of gamma photons, the annihilation event is known to have occurred along the line joining the two detectors. Raw PET scan data consist of a number of these coincidence lines, which are reorganized in to projections that identify where activity is concentrated within the patient. The utility of PET is based not only on its sensitivity but also on the fact that the most commonly used radionuclides (^{11}C, ^{13}N, ^{15}O, ^{18}F) are isotopes of elements that occur naturally in organic molecule. Although fluorine does not technically fit in to this category, it is a chemical substitute for hydrogen.

SPECT IN TMJ

A long bore fan beam collimator for imaging the head was designed and constructed for a SPECT system with a rotating scintillation camera. In order to avoid the patient's shoulder during rotation of the camera with thick camera housing, the long bore design is necessary to allow the collimator to get close to the patient's head for improved spatial resolution. Operating at the minimum radius of rotation, the prototype fan beam collimator provides about the same spatial resolution as the high resolution collimator, while the geometric efficiency is equal to approximately 85% of that of the general purpose and approximately 55% higher than the high resolution collimator. Images from a phantom study demonstrate good image quality and are void of artifacts. Comparative clinical studies between the LEGP and fan beam collimators also confirm the superior image quality obtained with the fan beam collimator.

Prospective evaluation by magnetic resonance imaging (MRI) and both single photon emission computed tomography (SPECT) and planar bone scintigraphy was undertaken by AZ Krasnow et al. They reported that the sensitivity of bone SPECT scintigraphy was 94%, arthrography was 96%, and planar bone scintigraphy was 76% compared with a 35% sensitivity of radionuclide angiography and 0.4% sensitivity of transcranial lateral radiographs. Bone SPECT exhibited significantly higher sensitivity than radionuclide angiography or transcranial lateral radiographs. A diagnostic sensitivity of 0.96 was achieved when the results of either MRI or SPECT was considered evidence of internal joint derangement. SPECT may be detecting functionally significant altered joint mechanics that are not evident on anatomic imaging of the TMJ.

Bone scintigraphy may be valuable to assess progress of TMJ inflammation or remodelling, and may affect diagnosis and treatment of patients with TMJ tenderness. The use of bone scintigraphy (bone scan) in the diagnosis of temporomandibular joint (TMJ) disease has been infrequent, as compared with traditional radiographic techniques. Bone scans have the potential to detect active bone remodelling whereas corresponding radiographs may be normal or document past structural change in the joint. Traditional radiographic findings and relevant clinical signs and symptoms correlated with bone scans may aid in the diagnosis of TMJ disease and possibly affect treatment and prognosis of individual cases. The use of bone scans as an additional tool in diagnosing TMJ disease was assessed in this series of patients by Epstein, Rea and Chahal.

Oesterreich et al performed semiquantitative SPECT imaging for assessment of bone reactions in internal derangements of the temporomandibular joint. They said that semi quantitative SPECT of the TMJs provides important information on the extent of osseous changes in afflicted joints and is suitable for follow-up of splint therapy. It may also be helpful as a screening method in detecting clinically normal joints before arthrography is carried out and in assessing the presumptive response to treatment with a splint.

Recently a study was undertaken by Coutinho A et al for the evaluation of single photon emission computed tomography with technetium 99m methylene diphosphonate (SPECT with 99mTc-MDP) and computed tomography (CT), simultaneously acquired image in diagnosis of temporomandibular joint (TMJ) dysfunction. A prospective study was conducted with 33 patients, 29 female and 4 male, all of them presenting signs and/or complaints suggestive of temporomandibular dysfunction. SPECT/CT with 99mTc-MDP was performed in all patients and imaging results compared with final diagnosis and clinical outcome. The correlation of signs and symptoms with SPECT/CT imaging showed sensitivity 100%, specificity 90.91%, and accuracy 96.97%. It was concluded that SPECT/CT with 99mTc-MDP co-registered imaging fusion is a suitable method of temporomandibular dysfunction diagnosis, due to the sensitivity, specificity, and accuracy observed.

BIBLIOGRAPHY

1. Aufdemorte TB, Van Sickels JE, Dolwick MF, et al. Estrogen receptors in the temporomandibular joint of the baboon: an autoradiographic study. Oral Surg Oral Med Oral Pathol 1986; 61:307–14.
2. AZ Krasnow, BD Collier, JB Kneeland, GF Carrera, DE Ryan, D Gingrass, S Sewall, RS Hellman, AT Isitman, W Froncisz. Comparison of high resolution MRI and SPECT bone scintigraphy for noninvasive imaging of the temporomandibular joint. J Nucl Med 1987;28(8):1268–74.
3. BM Tsui, GT Gullberg, ER Edgerton, DR Gilland, JR Perry, WH McCartney. Design and utility of a fan beam collimator for SPECT imaging of head. Journal of Nuclear Medicne 1986;27:6810–19.
4. Coutinho A, Fenyo-Pereira M, Dib LL, Lima EN. The role of SPECT/CT with 99mTc-MDP image fusion to diagnose temporomandibular dysfunction. Oral Surg Oral Med Oral Pathol Endod 2006; 101 (2): 224–30.
5. JB Epstein, A Rea, O Chahal. The use of bone scintigraphy in temporomandibular joint disorders. Oral Diseases 2002;8:47.
6. Oesterreich FU, Jend-Rossmann I. Jend HH. Triebel HJ. Semi-quantitative SPECT imaging for assessment of bone reactions in internal derangements of the temporomandibular joint. J Oral Maxillofac Surg 1987; 45(12):1022–8.
7. White & Pharaoh. Oral Radiology, Principles and interpretation. 5th Edition, pp 245–64.

Index

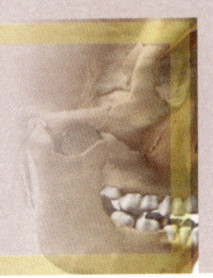

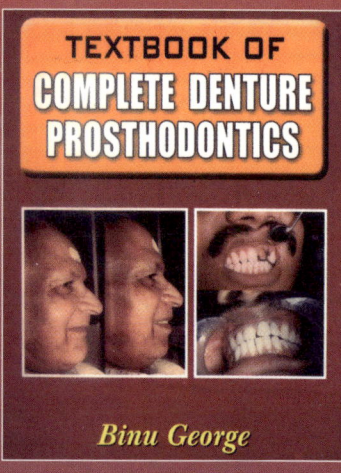

TEXTBOOK OF COMPLETE DENTURE PROSTHODONTICS

Binu George

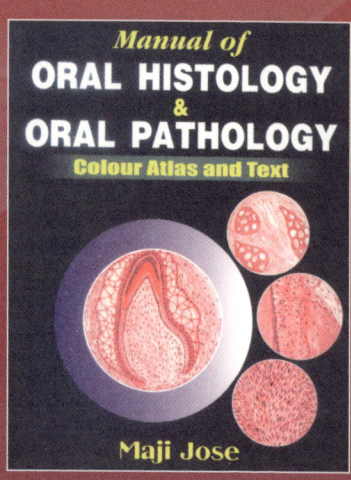

Manual of ORAL HISTOLOGY & ORAL PATHOLOGY
Colour Atlas and Text

Maji Jose

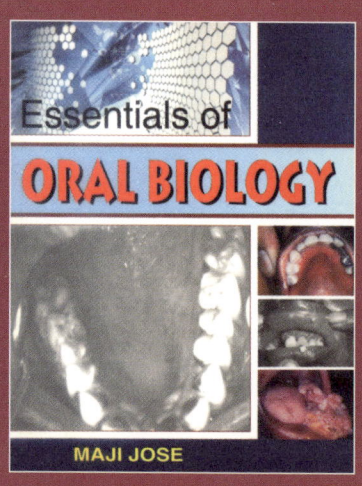

Essentials of **ORAL BIOLOGY**

MAJI JOSE

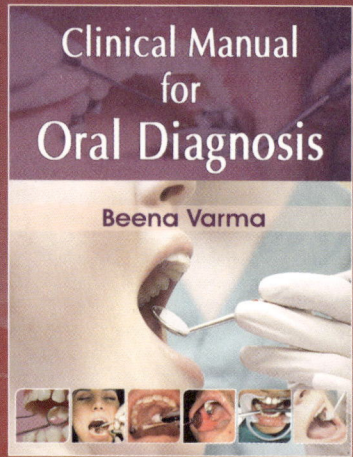

Clinical Manual for Oral Diagnosis

Beena Varma

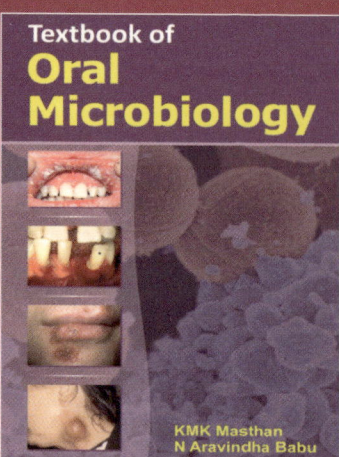

Textbook of **Oral Microbiology**

KMK Masthan
N Aravindha Babu